Telemedicine for the Musculoskeletal Physical Exam

Mariam Zakhary
Grant Cooper · Joseph Herrera
Editors

Telemedicine for the Musculoskeletal Physical Exam

A Pocket Guide

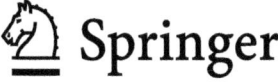

Editors
Mariam Zakhary
Department of Rehabilitation Medicine
Mount Sinai Hospital
New York, NY, USA

Grant Cooper
Princeton Spine and Joint Center
Princeton, NJ, USA

Joseph Herrera
Department of Rehabilitation Medicine
Mount Sinai Hospital
New York, NY, USA

ISBN 978-3-031-16872-7   ISBN 978-3-031-16873-4 (eBook)
https://doi.org/10.1007/978-3-031-16873-4

© The Editor(s) (if applicable) and The Author(s), under exclusive license to Springer Nature Switzerland AG 2023
This work is subject to copyright. All rights are solely and exclusively licensed by the Publisher, whether the whole or part of the material is concerned, specifically the rights of translation, reprinting, reuse of illustrations, recitation, broadcasting, reproduction on microfilms or in any other physical way, and transmission or information storage and retrieval, electronic adaptation, computer software, or by similar or dissimilar methodology now known or hereafter developed.
The use of general descriptive names, registered names, trademarks, service marks, etc. in this publication does not imply, even in the absence of a specific statement, that such names are exempt from the relevant protective laws and regulations and therefore free for general use.
The publisher, the authors, and the editors are safe to assume that the advice and information in this book are believed to be true and accurate at the date of publication. Neither the publisher nor the authors or the editors give a warranty, expressed or implied, with respect to the material contained herein or for any errors or omissions that may have been made. The publisher remains neutral with regard to jurisdictional claims in published maps and institutional affiliations.

This Springer imprint is published by the registered company Springer Nature Switzerland AG
The registered company address is: Gewerbestrasse 11, 6330 Cham, Switzerland

My incredible mother Amal and my late father and angel Adel. My partner in all things, my husband Bishoy. My biggest motivators, my brother George and his wife Marian, and my biggest fans, my nephews Noah and Jeremiah.
Mariam Zakhary

For Ana, Mila, Lara, Luka, Twinkle, and Lili
Grant Cooper

Acknowledgments

To my coeditors and to my authors—this isn't for you, but by you. Thank you. Dr. Herrera, you have been a friend, a mentor, and a guiding presence throughout my entire career, and I am honored to have completed this project with you. Thank you to my outstanding residents German and Craig who kept this machine going and were my right-hand men. Thank you to my husband Bishoy who has had to deal with my highs and lows throughout the process and made sure the lows were outnumbered. Your patience exceeds any and all expectations—you're the real MVP.
Mariam Zakhary

It has been a pleasure to collaborate on this book. I want to first thank my coeditors and all of the amazing authors who worked so hard to make this book a reality. In particular to my good friend and colleague, Dr. Herrera, it's great to finish yet another terrific project with you. Thank you to my colleagues at Princeton Spine & Joint Center for continuing to push, nurture, and challenge me. And thank you to my family, Ana, Mila, Lara, Luka, Twinkle, and Lili, for putting up with me when I disappeared into the study to write.
Grant Cooper

I would like to thank my amazing family, Sandra, Alex, Mikhayla, and Andrew, for all of their continued love and support through this journey. Thank you to all of our fantastic authors and other editors who came together to make this book a success.
Joseph Herrera

Contents

1. **Remote Patient Monitoring** 1
   David Putrino, Tina Bijlani, Jenna M. Tosto-Mancuso, and Laura Tabacof

2. **Video Visit Preparation and Patient Education** 17
   Aaron Bolds and Amanda A. Kelly

3. **The General Telemedicine Exam** 23
   Elinor H. Naor

4. **The Telemedicine Cervical Spine Exam** 39
   Chandni Patel, Jonathan Ramin, and David A. Spinner

5. **The Telemedicine Thoracic Spine Exam** 49
   David A. Spinner, Caroline Alyse Varlotta, and Alexandra Laurent

6. **The Telemedicine Lumbar Spine Exam** 67
   Rebecca Freedman, Jonathan Lee, and David A. Spinner

7. **The Telemedicine Shoulder Exam** 81
   Mariam Zakhary, Craig Silverberg, and Angela Samaan

8. **The Telemedicine Elbow Exam** 91
   Mariam Zakhary, German Valdez, and Monica Gibilisco

9	**The Telemedicine Hand and Wrist Exam** 105
	Andres Arredondo, Hashem E. Zikry, and Amie M. Kim

10	**The Telemedicine Hip Exam** 125
	Jasmin Harounian, Carley Trentman, and Richard G. Chang

11	**The Telemedicine Knee Exam** 135
	Michelle N. Leong, Laurenie G. Louissaint, and Joseph Herrera

12	**The Telemedicine Foot and Ankle Exam**. 159
	Christopher Clifford, Liam J. Rawson, Lissa Hewan-Lowe, and Amie M. Kim

13	**Telemedicine Evaluation and Management of Respiratory Muscle Dysfunction**. 183
	Michael Chiou, John R. Bach, and Charles Kent

14	**The Telemedicine Functional Assessment**. 195
	Joseph Herrera, Andrew Beaufort, and Kaitlyn E. Wilkey

Index. 215

Contributors

Andres Arredondo, MD Department of Emergency Medicine, Icahn School of Medicine at Mount Sinai, New York, NY, USA

John R. Bach, MD Department of Physical Medicine and Rehabilitation, Rutgers New Jersey Medical School, Newark, NJ, USA

Andrew Beaufort, MD Department of Rehabilitation and Human Performance, Icahn School of Medicine at Mount Sinai, New York, NY, USA

Tina Bijlani, DO Department of Rehabilitation and Human Performance, Icahn School of Medicine at Mount Sinai, New York, NY, USA

Aaron Bolds, MD Department of Rehabilitation and Human Performance, Mount Sinai Hospital, New York, NY, USA

Richard G. Chang, MD Department of Rehabilitation and Human Performance, Icahn School of Medicine at Mount Sinai, New York, NY, USA

Michael Chiou, MD Department of Rehabilitation and Human Performance, Icahn School of Medicine at Mount Sinai, New York, NY, USA

Christopher Clifford, MD Department of Emergency Medicine, Mount Sinai Icahn School of Medicine, New York, NY, USA

Rebecca Freedman, DO Department of Rehabilitation and Human Performance, Mount Sinai Hospital, New York, NY, USA

Monica Gibilisco, DO Department of Rehabilitation and Human Performance, Mount Sinai Hospital, New York, NY, USA

Jasmin Harounian, MD Department of Rehabilitation and Human Performance, Icahn School of Medicine at Mount Sinai, New York, NY, USA

Joseph Herrera, DO Department of Rehabilitation and Human Performance, Icahn School of Medicine, Mount Sinai Hospital, New York, NY, USA

Department of Rehabilitation and Human Performance, Mount Sinai Hospital, New York, NY, USA

Lissa Hewan-Lowe, DO Department of Physical Medicine Rehabilitation, Mount Sinai Icahn School of Medicine, New York, NY, USA

Amanda A. Kelly, MD Department of Rehabilitation and Human Performance, Mount Sinai Hospital, New York, NY, USA

Charles Kent, DO Department of Rehabilitation and Human Performance, Icahn School of Medicine at Mount Sinai, New York, NY, USA

Amie M. Kim, MD Department of Emergency Medicine, Department of Physical Medicine Rehabilitation, Icahn School of Medicine at Mount Sinai at Beth Israel, New York, NY, USA

Alexandra Laurent, DO Department of Rehabilitation and Human Performance, Mount Sinai Hospital, Scarsdale, NY, USA

Jonathan Lee, DO Department of Rehabilitation and Human Performance, Mount Sinai Hospital, New York, NY, USA

Michelle N. Leong, DO Department of Rehabilitation and Human Performance, Icahn School of Medicine, Mount Sinai Hospital, New York, NY, USA

Laurenie G. Louissaint, MD Department of Rehabilitation and Human Performance, Icahn School of Medicine, Mount Sinai Hospital, New York, NY, USA

Elinor H. Naor, DO Department of Physical Medicine and Rehabilitation, Mount Sinai Hospital, New York, NY, USA

Chandni Patel, DO Department of Rehabilitation and Human Performance, Icahn School of Medicine at Mount Sinai, New York, NY, USA

David Putrino, PT, PhD Department of Rehabilitation and Human Performance, Icahn School of Medicine at Mount Sinai, New York, NY, USA

Jonathan Ramin, DO Department of Rehabilitation and Human Performance, Icahn School of Medicine at Mount Sinai, New York, NY, USA

Liam J. Rawson, MD Department of Emergency Medicine, Mount Sinai Morningside/West, New York, NY, USA

Angela Samaan, DO Department of Rehabilitation and Human Performance, Icahn School of Medicine at Mount Sinai, New York, NY, USA

Craig Silverberg, DO Department of Rehabilitation and Human Performance, Icahn School of Medicine at Mount Sinai, New York, NY, USA

David A. Spinner, DO Department of Rehabilitation and Human Performance, Icahn School of Medicine at Mount Sinai, New York, NY, USA

Department of Rehabilitation and Human Performance, Mount Sinai Hospital, New York, NY, USA

Laura Tabacof, MD Department of Rehabilitation and Human Performance, Icahn School of Medicine at Mount Sinai, New York, NY, USA

Jenna M. Tosto-Mancuso, DPT Department of Rehabilitation and Human Performance, Icahn School of Medicine at Mount Sinai, New York, NY, USA

Carley Trentman, MD Department of Rehabilitation and Human Performance, Icahn School of Medicine at Mount Sinai, New York, NY, USA

German Valdez, MD Department of Rehabilitation and Human Performance, Mount Sinai Hospital, New York, NY, USA

Caroline Alyse Varlotta, DO Department of Rehabilitation and Human Performance, Mount Sinai Hospital, Scarsdale, NY, USA

Kaitlyn E. Wilkey, DO Department of Rehabilitation and Human Performance, Icahn School of Medicine at Mount Sinai, New York, NY, USA

Mariam Zakhary, DO Department of Rehabilitation and Human Performance, Icahn School of Medicine at Mount Sinai, New York, NY, USA

Department of Rehabilitation Medicine, Mount Sinai Hospital, New York, NY, USA

Hashem E. Zikry, MD Department of Emergency Medicine, Icahn School of Medicine at Mount Sinai, New York, NY, USA

Remote Patient Monitoring

David Putrino, Tina Bijlani,
Jenna M. Tosto-Mancuso, and Laura Tabacof

Remote Patient Monitoring (RPM): Working Definition and Central Concepts

Remote patient monitoring is a form of *home-based telehealth* that enables patient monitoring and transfer of physiological and clinical data to healthcare providers to assist in clinical management and decision-making. In RPM systems, data can be acquired and transmitted by a range of platforms: from mobile applications to peripheral measurement devices (blood pressure cuffs and pulse oximeters) and modern wearable biosensors (integrated into smartphones, watches, wristbands, shoes, or textiles). RPM systems can also transmit user-entered data and include video interaction and real-time chat with clinical providers. Health data is transmitted to remote care providers, either in real-time (*synchronous* or "real time interactive systems") or intermittently (*asynchronous* or "store and forward"), and it can be stored in secure health records for clinical review, interpreta-

---

D. Putrino (✉) · T. Bijlani · J. M. Tosto-Mancuso · L. Tabacof
Department of Rehabilitation and Human Performance, Icahn School of Medicine at Mount Sinai, New York, NY, USA
e-mail: david.putrino@mountsinai.org; jenna.tosto@mountsinai.org; laura.tabacof@mountsinai.org

© The Author(s), under exclusive license to Springer Nature Switzerland AG 2023
M. Zakhary et al. (eds.), *Telemedicine for the Musculoskeletal Physical Exam*, https://doi.org/10.1007/978-3-031-16873-4_1

tion, and intervention. RPM systems can also be designed to flag abnormalities and alert providers, who can review the data to provide clinical guidance, schedule a follow-up visit or advise escalation of care (indicating a hospital or emergency room visit).

RPM is typically deployed after hospital discharge or between routine office visits, allowing clinicians to monitor daily vitals and symptoms between formal healthcare visits and reinforce post-discharge instructions. By closing the gap in patient management, RPM allows the possibility for early intervention and improved clinical management, reducing healthcare utilization and associated costs [1, 2].

The Value of RPM in Telemedicine

In the last decades, with the rapid development of telemedicine, RPM has emerged as a promising modality. RPM features benefits which are common to other telehealth approaches including the potential to expand healthcare accessibility for individuals living in rural or isolated areas [3], optimize healthcare services [3] and decrease healthcare costs. However, one of the most unique features of RPM that differentiates it from other telehealth modalities is the ability to leverage technological innovation to enhance healthcare delivery. Deploying wearable sensors allow continuous gathering of longitudinal physiological data which can assist in clinical management and decision-making to optimize healthcare assistance. In addition, it provides abundant data for research and advances further understanding of disease physiology and symptomatology [3]. Also, due to RPM's asynchronous features, providers are spared from actively collecting data and can therefore spend more time and effort in treatment and education of patients, potentially increasing work productivity and efficiency. Moreover, the use of bidirectional features (including real-time chat with clinical providers) allows RPM to have a uniquely human feature, giving patients a feeling of reassurance. In addition, giving patients clinical feedback has the potential to empower them with their own data, giving them the ability to take ownership of their condition and assume a more active role in their treatment, which can be particularly relevant for chronic health conditions where disease control (and not treatment per se) is the main focus.

Initially, the primary application of RPM was in clinical management of chronic diseases such as diabes, hypertension, asthma, and COPD [1, 4, 5]. By providing disease-specific patient education (i.e., how to recognize symptom exacerbation and what symptoms require clinical intervention) and guiding self-management best practice (by optimizing medication intake, dietary, and lifestyle guidance), RPM shows promising results to improve health-related outcomes in patients with COPD, Parkinson's, hypertension, and low back pain [2]. Multiple types of interventions have been deployed and the ones based on health behavior models and personalized coaching appear to be the most successful and achieved greater clinical results. Overall, RPM interventions are well accepted by patients and show high levels of compliance and engagement [1, 5, 6, 7]. They are capable of reducing hospital readmission (with significant cost savings) and improve participants' self-efficacy in disease management and control [1].

Over time, RPM has expanded its role and was shown to be feasible, engaging, and beneficial in the fields of postpartum [7], post-operative surgery [8, 9], weight management, and elderly care [10, 11]. More recently, the role of RPM during the COVID-19 world pandemic has received new attention. Its asynchronous and bidirectional features [3] allows mass-scale screening and patient management in a de-hospitalized fashion, decompressing the healthcare system and avoiding face-to face interactions that might further spread the virus. For its unique features and operational characteristics, RPM is a promising tool to enhance patient outcomes in a cost-effective and scalable manner.

RPM and MSK: Introduction

Musculoskeletal disorders are widespread and one of the most common complaints experienced by patients. During extenuating circumstances such as the COVID-19 pandemic, patients were unable to be seen face to face, as providers were unavailable or clinics were closed. Remote patient monitoring can provide a unique way for patients to receive care for one of the most common conditions.

By definition, telemedicine is the use of communication technologies to provide patient care when patients and clinicians are physically distanced [12]. While telemedicine has evolved to allow individuals with a variety of diagnoses to meet with a medical provider remotely using video or telephonic systems, remote patient monitoring has grown to further increase the health system's capacity to provide care remotely. Remote patient monitoring, or RPM encompasses the remote evaluation of physiologic data transmitted from the patient to the health system via technology. The capacity for remote patient monitoring can be especially helpful in providing comprehensive care to patients with musculoskeletal injuries as it allows for increased follow-up, improved communication between patients and healthcare providers, and more frequent assessment to further inform clinical decision-making and optimize patient care.

Remote patient monitoring systems function to obtain physiologic data from patients using measurable, quantifiable metrics. It has historically been used to obtain data from electrocardiograms (ECG), electroencephalogram (EEG), heart rate, respiratory rate, pulse oximetry, blood pressure, body temperature, and blood glucose levels [13].

Extrapolating on this data to apply to the musculoskeletal patient will allow increased access to health care for patients with common musculoskeletal disorders. It will also allow them to be monitored continuously with faster and convenient care while effectively reducing hospital costs. With the advent of RPM for monitoring patients with cardiopulmonary disease and those with dermatologic and stroke conditions, one should explore its utility in other fields of medicine.

Remote patient monitoring and the field of telemedicine is believed to have started in the 1960s under projects initiated by the National Aeronautics and Space Administration (NASA) [14]. As NASA expanded investigation into the physiological barriers and implications of space flight on the human body, the need to assess the cardiovascular and respiratory systems arose. To evaluate these medical quandaries, animal subjects were the first known users of remote patient monitoring studies. Animal subjects were sent on test flights to space while physiologic data was remotely captured by scientists on Earth (NASA) [14]. As the program further developed, this form of remote patient monitoring further evolved to include the physiologic data monitoring of astronaut's mid space flight [15]. Since then, the face of telemedicine, and particularly remote patient monitoring, has vastly changed given the advent of novel technology and the seamless integration of technology into modern medical practice. RPM has been utilized in a variety of diagnoses including but not limited to individuals with neurological, cardiovascular, respiratory, orthopedic. Current RPM models include a variety of patient populations as detailed above. While the literature examining the clinical utility of remote patient monitoring in the musculoskeletal patient continues to evolve, this presents as an exciting opportunity for further development of the RPM space.

Remote Patient Monitoring for the Musculoskeletal Patient

Musculoskeletal conditions are characterized by pain, limitations in mobility, and decreased function, affecting the joints, bones, muscles, ligaments, and tendons of the body. Persistent pain caused by these conditions can limit a patients' ability to participate in social roles, limit dexterity, and functional ability at work. The consequences include and are not limited to decreased participation in the community, reduced quality of life, and poor mental well-being (report on the impact of MSK EU citation).

Musculoskeletal pain was reported to be one of the leading causes of disability, according to the Global Burden of Disease studies (GBD). Half of the adult population has reported to experience musculoskeletal symptoms and 39–45% will have persistent symptoms [16]. Musculoskeletal conditions have periods of remission and exacerbation, and therefore patients do not always experience full resolution of symptoms, requiring consistent medical attention.

The etiology of musculoskeletal pathology includes inflammation, wear-and-tear, overuse, and secondary to acute injury. These can most commonly affect the shoulder, elbow, wrist, hand, digit, spine, hip, knee, foot, and ankle. In the traditional office setting, patients present with a chief complaint. Next, a detailed history is obtained by the clinician. Patients are evaluated as a whole unit with special attention to the affected body part. The first part of the examination includes assessing for erythema, swelling, asymmetry, and bony deformities. A joint examination is performed where the range of motion is assessed and compared to normal values in order to evaluate for restriction or pathology. A manual muscle strength examination and deep tendon reflex test is performed. Additionally, the clinician will evaluate for falls, gait, posture, and a comprehensive functional evaluation.

Remote patient monitoring for the musculoskeletal patient can be a valuable tool for the physical medicine and rehabilitation physician and other similar specialists. The advancement of technology with innovative wearable devices and smartphone applications allows for faster data transmission and improved standardization from patient to clinician. Not only can this technology be used to diagnose and monitor patients, but it can also be used to implement a rehabilitation treatment plan. To provide health care to patients who do not have the means or access, remote patient monitoring can be instrumental in providing quality care while alleviating these debilitating musculoskeletal conditions. Here we will present examples for metrics that can be remotely monitored by the rehabilitation physician.

Inspection

During a clinical visit the patients' affected body part can be visualized in real time. With the advent of RPM, patients can send photos of images for conditions that require monitoring. For example, a patient with erythema, edema, and/or ecchymosis can be remotely monitored by sending images to their healthcare provider. This should be compared to the contralateral body part, noting changes in shape, size, color, or structural differences. Multiple images provide additional data points and can be superior to the traditional office visit when the provider only sees the patients at the initial and follow-up visits.

Pain

Pain monitoring is important to understand the severity of a patient's symptoms and should be included in the RPM platform. It has been used in remote patient monitoring applications historically. In the Keele Pain recorder feasibility study, Bedson et al. demonstrated the use of an application to monitor painful musculoskeletal conditions in response to analgesic prescribing [17]. Using the VAS scale in a questionnaire format, patients can document their pain level on a scale from 0 (no pain) to 10 (worst pain). To obtain a more accurate, in-depth pain assessment, the questionnaire should include onset (acute or gradual), qualitative factors, course over time (constant or intermittent), and impact on functional status. Provoking and alleviating factors should be recorded, as well as comparison between pain levels at rest versus with activity. Additionally qualitative factors that differentiate nociceptive from neuropathic pain are important and should be addressed. Questions to be included in the RPM questionnaire include listing if the pain feels more like a shooting, burning, or stabbing pain, associated with paresthesias, which is more indicative of neuropathic pain.

Range of Motion

Depending on the location of pain, the specific joint should be assessed for flexion, extension, abduction, internal rotation, and/or external rotation, and this should be compared to the contralateral side. In the office passive range of motion can be compared to active range of motion. Passive range of motion is assessed when the examiner takes the joint to the end range of motion, while active range of motion is examined when the patient moves to their limit of motion without assistance. Range of motion can be limited by several types of pathology including contractures and spasticity.

Ramkumar et al. [8, 9] evaluated the utility in RPM for patients after total knee arthroplasty with favorable results indicating that RPM can evaluate patients' mobility and rehabilitation compliance. A wearable knee sleeve with Velcro straps and Bluetooth-enabled sensors transmitted positional data directly to the smartphone for machine learning analysis and real-time display of ROM. This was found to be effective when evaluating active range of motion of the knee by prompting patients to determine maximum flexion with heel slide. This type of technology can be translated to other joints of the body and can provide clinicians increased data points about range of motion limitations that may indicate pathology.

Palpation

Palpation is notably limited with the RPM assessment; however, patients' self-reports of tenderness should be included and can be indicative of pathology. For example, bicipital groove tenderness can be associated with bicipital tendinitis. Within the RPM platform, the patient should be able to click to points of painful palpation.

Strength

Evaluating manual muscle strength (manual muscle test) is integral to the musculoskeletal examination. Patterns of weakness can localize a lesion to the nerve root, peripheral nerve, or specific muscle. Similarly to examination above, the strength of each muscle should be recorded with the contralateral side to assess for asymmetry. Muscle strength is rated on a grading scale from 0 to 5.

Grade	Muscle response
0	No contraction detected
1	Barely detectable flicker or trace of contraction
2	Active movement with gravity eliminated
3	Active movement against gravity
4	Active movement against gravity and with some resistance
5	Active movement against resistance, "normal"

A caretaker can be trained to perform the MMT assessment with the specific grading system above. When patients live alone or do not have the help of a caretaker, household objects can be utilized to assess strength. If able to be obtained, a dynamometer can assess hand grip strength.

Lower extremity muscle activation against gravity can be assessed at home and recorded into an RPM platform. The double leg squat and rise can be utilized to evaluate quadriceps and lower extremity strength. The single leg sit to stand test to assess for more subtle quad weakness, which is important in evaluating patients with L3–L4 radiculopathy. Additionally, patients can walk on their heels and toes to evaluate for L5 and S1 weakness, respectively. Weakness with repetitive toe raises can indicate more subtle S1 weakness [18].

Sensation

Sensation is an important aspect of the musculoskeletal examination when testing for neurologic deficits. In the office setting, the examiner will evaluate the patient's ability to feel light touch and pain/sharp/pinprick while comparing both sides. Light touch is tested with a cotton wisp whereas pain sensation can be tested using a pin. Similarly to the self-reported palpation for tenderness above, patients can self-report loss or changes in sensation in a questionnaire format.

Function and Mobility

Functional mobility is the manner in which patients can move around in their environment in order to participate in activities of daily living. Function and mobility are important components of the musculoskeletal evaluation. A metric to evaluate mobility is the gait speed. Specialized sensors such as the Moterum Application [19] can measure important aspects of the gait cycle including walking speed, stride time variability, stance time/symmetry, and step time/symmetry with the goal to enhance patients' gait. Smartphone applications with self-administering applications to assess gait instability have been developed [20]. The Timed Up and Go Test (iTUG) and the 30-second chair stand test (30s-CST) have been developed for android phones and iPhones. Some applications can distinguish between sit-to-stand and stand-to-sit subphases of the chair stand test [20] or the sit-to-stand, walk, turn, walk, stand-to-sit subphases of the iTUG test.

Technology Utilized in RPM

Technological advances have facilitated data capture and data transmission for remote physiologic monitoring in the RPM space. While a breadth of literature exists to explore the utilization of RPM in pioneers of RPM programming such as cardiology, technological adaptation for physiologic monitoring continues to grow in the musculoskeletal space. Wearable devices and smart garments continue to gain increasing popularity with both clinicians and patients alike. In a recent review by Porciuncula et al., numerous wearable devices have been identified in the literature as viable options for remote patient monitoring and telehealth use [21]. Digital accelerometers, gyroscopes, and force sensors are commonly implemented to capture gait metrics including stride length, ground reaction forces, and acceleration/deceleration forces. In patients with knee osteoarthritis and those following total knee replacement, kinematic analysis of range of motion and knee kinematics throughout functional mobility have been shown to be reliable indicators of mobility, physical activity, and range of motion. Additionally, utilization of RPM data collection can allow for optimal care of performance athletes, including runners, to better understand gait mechanics for optimize clinical decision-making in running-related injuries. Biomechanical data collection collected over RPM has the capacity to optimize clinical decision-making across musculoskeletal management [22].

When to Triage for Telemedicine or Video Visit

Red flag symptoms can be remotely documented, including those indicative of pain due to cancer, acute injury requiring urgent attention, or pain that is secondary to a non-musculoskeletal etiology. For example, when evaluating low back pain, questions should be asked to evaluate if patients have pain caused by tumor, infection, spinal fracture, or major neurologic compromise, such as cauda equina syndrome.

Barriers of RPM

The tactile sensory and palpatory aspect of the musculoskeletal examination can be difficult with the RPM platform. Ways to circumvent this reliance on a second examiner, such as utilizing a wearable device, can come with prohibitive costs or may require complex programming code to process the data.

An important aspect with RPM includes physiologic data tracking. When technology cannot accurately assess and/or match up with a physiologic symptom, it limits the clinicians' ability to get a comprehensive evaluation of the patient. Additionally, this technology excludes patients without the ability to read and understand the language, patients who may have cognitive deficits, or those with limited access to technology.

Billing and Coding Legislation

While the advent of RPM has allowed for expansion and modernization of healthcare practice with a myriad of benefits, several notable barriers in both institutional, professional, and patient centered domains need to be addressed in order to successfully integrate an RPM program into clinical practice [23].

Established in 2019 and finalized to become more readily accessible in January of 2020, Centers for Medicare and Medicaid Services (CMS) established a novel set of Current Procedural Terminology (CPT) codes to be utilized for the chronic remote monitoring of pre-established physiologic parameters [24]. There has been a strict enforcement on the appropriate physiologic measures being monitored and the way in which data is transmitted and shared through a remote device. In order for a remote patient monitoring service rendered to be successfully reimbursed, CMS has clarified strict criteria that all RPM services should meet. Such criteria includes that all devices used to collect physiologic data must electronically automatically collect and transmit data, i.e., automatically [24]. Furthermore, the device must be defined as a Section 201(h) device by the Federal Food, Drug, and Cosmetic Act (FD&C) [25]. This may present a barrier for device selection and implementation as it requires both the end user (patient) and clinician utilizing have access to a Smart Device enabled with an application programming interface (API). API allows for the transmission.

Additional reimbursement barriers faced while implementing a remote patient monitoring program include the required number of clinical data encounters required to successfully bill the implementation and data monitoring CPT codes (99453, 99454). CMS requires that at least 16 data encounters are recorded over the course of 30 days for the CPT codes to be appropriately billed. For patients who are less technologically savvy or for those with chronic conditions requiring intermittent monitoring may report fewer episodes and thus the provider may be unable to successfully be reimbursed for the above identified codes [24].

References

1. De San Miguel K, Smith J, Lewin G. Telehealth remote monitoring for community-dwelling older adults with chronic obstructive pulmonary disease. Telemed. J. E. Health. 2013;19:652–57. https://doi.org/10.1089/tmj.2012.0244. [PubMed].
2. Noah B, Keller MS, Mosadeghi S et al. Impact of remote patient monitoring on clinical outcomes: an updated meta-analysis of randomized controlled trials. NPJ Digit Med. 2018;1:20172. https://doi.org/10.1038/s41746-017-0002-4.
3. Watson AR, Wah R, Thamman R. The value of remote monitoring for the COVID-19 pandemic. Telemed J E Health. 2020;26(9):1110–2.
4. Stone RA, Rao RH, Sevick MA, Cheng C, Hough LJ, Macpherson DS, et al. Active care management supported by home telemonitoring in veterans with type 2 diabetes: the DiaTel randomized controlled trial. Diabetes Care. 2010;33(3):478–84.
5. AbuDagga A, Resnick HE, Alwan M. Impact of blood pressure telemonitoring on hypertension outcomes: a literature review. Telemed J E Health. 2010;16(7):830–8.

6. Ginis P, Nieuwboer A, Dorfman M, Ferrari A, Gazit E, Canning CG, et al. Feasibility and effects of home-based smartphone-delivered automated feedback training for gait in people with Parkinson's disease: a pilot randomized controlled trial. Parkinsonism Relat Disord. 2016;22:2834.
   Hauspurg A, Lemon L, Quinn BA, Binstock A, Larkin J, Beigi RH, Watson AR, Hyagriv SN. A postpartum remote hypertension monitoring protocol implemented at the hospital level. Obstetrics & Gynecology. 2019;134(4):685–91. https://doi.org/10.1097/AOG.0000000000003479.
7. Ramkumar PN, Haeberle HS, Ramanathan D, Cantrell WA, Navarro SM, Mont MA, et al. Remote patient monitoring using mobile health for total knee arthroplasty: validation of a wearable and machine learning-based surveillance platform. J Arthroplasty. 2019;34(10):2253–9.
8. Ramkumar PN, Haeberle HS, Bloomfield MR, Schaffer JL, Kamath AF, Patterson BM, et al. Artificial intelligence and arthroplasty at a single institution: real-world applications of machine learning to big data, value-based care, mobile health, and remote patient monitoring. J Arthroplasty. 2019;34(10):2204–9.
9. Hong E, Jakacic AN, Sahoo A, Breyman E, Ukegbu G, Tabacof L, et al. Use of Fitbit technology does not impact health biometrics in a community of older adults. Telemed J E Health. 2020;27(4):409–13.
10. Hamilton T, Johnson L, Quinn BT, Coppola J, Sachs D, Migliaccio J, et al. Telehealth intervention programs for seniors: an observational study of a community-embedded health monitoring initiative. Telemed J E Health. 2020;26(4):438–45.
11. Field MJ, Grigsby J. Telemedicine and remote patient monitoring. JAMA. 2002;288(4):423–5.
12. Malasinghe LP, Ramzan N, Dahal K. Remote patient monitoring: a comprehensive study. J Ambient Intell Humaniz Comput. 2017;10(1):57–76.
13. NASA. Updated October 4 2020. https://www.nasa.gov/content/a-brief-history-of-nasa-s-contributions-totelemedicine#_ednref1. Accessed 12 Oct 2020.
14. Doarn CR, Nicogossian AE, Merrell RC. Applications of telemedicine in the United States space program. Telemed J. 1998;4(1):19–30.
15. James SL, Abate D, Abate KH, Abay SM, Abbafati C, Abbasi N, et al. Global, regional, and national incidence, prevalence, and years lived with disability for 354 diseases and injuries for 195 countries and territories, 1990–2017: a systematic analysis for the Global Burden of Disease Study 2017. Lancet. 2018;392(10159):1789–858.
16. Bedson J, Hill J, White D, Chen Y, Wathall S, Dent S, et al. Development and validation of a pain monitoring app for patients with musculoskeletal conditions (The Keele pain recorder feasibility study). BMC Med Inform Decis Mak. 2019;19(1):24.
17. Bergquist R, Vereijken B, Mellone S, Corzani M, Helbostad JL, Taraldsen K. App-based self-administrable clinical tests of physical function: development and usability study. JMIR Mhealth Uhealth. 2020;8(4):e16507.

18. Telemedicine: Here To Stay—Moterum Technologies. https://moterum.com/telemedicine-here-to-stay/.
19. Blair CK, Harding E, Herman C, Boyce T, Demark-Wahnefried W, Davis S, et al. Remote assessment of functional mobility and strength in older cancer survivors: protocol for a validity and reliability study. JMIR Res Protoc. 2020;9(9):e20834.
20. Porciuncula F, Roto AV, Kumar D, Davis I, Roy S, Walsh CJ, et al. Wearable movement sensors for rehabilitation: a focused review of technological and clinical advances. PM R. 2018;10(9 Suppl 2):S220–S32.
21. Laskowski ER, Johnson SE, Shelerud RA, Lee JA, Rabatin AE, Driscoll SW, et al. The telemedicine musculoskeletal examination. Mayo Clin Proc. 2020;95(8):1715–31.
22. LeRouge C, Garfield MJ. Crossing the telemedicine chasm: have the U.S. barriers to widespread adoption of telemedicine been significantly reduced? Int J Environ Res Public Health. 2013;10(12):6472–84.
23. Clinical Medical Services. Updated 4 October 2020. https://www.cms.gov/newsroom/fact-sheets/proposed-policypayment-and-quality-provisions-changes-medicare-physician-fee-schedule-calendar-year-4. Accessed 12 Oct 2020.
24. U.S. Food and Drug Administration. Updated October 4th 2020. https://www.fda.gov/medical-devices/classify-yourmedical-device/how-determine-if-your-product-medical-device. Accessed 12 Oct 2020.

Video Visit Preparation and Patient Education

Aaron Bolds and Amanda A. Kelly

General Description

In this chapter, we will discuss how to best prepare a patient for a video visit. We will focus on important information to give to your patient in preparation for the visit and certain factors to consider when conducting a video visit.

Prior to the Visit

It is important to ensure that the patient understands and is agreeable to a video visit. Once this has been established, the patient should be given clear instructions on how to best prepare for the appointment in order to optimize time, space, and quality of the visit. Most importantly, instructions on how to connect to the telemedicine platform should be given to the patient several days before the appointment. This will ensure that the patient has time to download any applicable software and get familiarized with the controls; this will help to prevent time inefficiency [1]. Provider

A. Bolds (✉) · A. A. Kelly
Department of Rehabilitation and Human Performance, Mount Sinai Hospital, New York, NY, USA
e-mail: aaron.bolds@mountsinai.org; Amanda.Kelly@mountsinai.org

and staff training play an essential role in the preparation for the televisit. Providers and staff should conduct mock televisits amongst themselves to help identify potential obstacles [2]. This will ensure that providers, nursing staff, front desk staff, and others are familiar with how to prevent issues and troubleshoot in the event they occur.

Optimizing Visual and Auditory Quality

The visual and auditory quality of the video stream is very important to the visit. Advise the patient to choose a well-lit, quiet room, and ideally an area that will minimize the likelihood of family members or friends interrupting the appointment. The patient may ask for the assistance of another person to help manage the camera and adjust camera angles, which may be beneficial during the physical exam portion of the visit. Lastly, ask the patient to choose a space that has good internet connection to best prevent any technical disruptions during the appointment [3].

Choosing an Ideal Space

Given that the physical exam is a very important component of any musculoskeletal complaint, it is important that the patient be advised to choose a space that will allow for all necessary maneuvers. The patient should choose a large space that will allow for full range of motion. The patient should keep in mind that they will likely have to sit, stand, lie down, and walk around in this area for a comprehensive physical exam. As the history-taking portion of the visit will likely take place sitting, the patient should prepare a chair in the room [3].

Clothing

In order to ensure that the patient is best able to perform all physical exam maneuvers, the patient should be instructed to wear comfortable, loose-fitting clothes. This can include athletic shorts, tank tops, or T-shirts.

Helpful Objects

It may be useful to instruct the patient to have several objects in the room that can be used during the physical exam portion of the visit. This can include household objects to provide resistance during muscle strength testing, or the patient may ask another person to provide resistance if he/she feels comfortable. A cotton swab may be used to test light touch and a safety pin may be used to test pin prick. Lastly, a flat-sided object such as a cell phone or book may be used for reflex testing [1].

During the Visit

At the start of the appointment, confirm the patient's identity and consent to move forward with the video visit. Then, give the patient an overview of what to expect. As with a regular visit, this will include identifying the chief complaint, obtaining the history of present illness or interval history, review of systems, physical exam, assessment/plan, and answering any questions [1]. At this point, continue to conduct the visit as you normally would a regular visit. Modifications to the physical exam portion of the visit can be made as described in subsequent chapters based on the affected area. It is important that documentation provides a description of the maneuvers used for physical exam since it will sometimes require improvisation.

After the Visit

Once the assessment and plan has been shared with the patient and all questions have been answered, check to see if the patient has access to their electronic chart. If not, be sure to find another method of providing the patient with an after-visit summary. This can be mail, email, or fax. Be sure to schedule appropriate follow-up with the patient, whether this be telemedicine or in-person.

Preparing Your Patient for the Video Visit/Patient Education

Outline

- Prior to appointment, ensure patient knows appointment is virtual.
- Prior to appointment, give patient clear instructions on how to optimize visual quality of visit, time, and space.
    - Give patients instructions on how to connect to telemedicine platform and test connection prior to the day of appointment. This can prevent time-wasting [1].
    - Patient should choose a well-lit, quiet room, with good internet connection, minimize likelihood of other family members entering space [3].
    - Patient should also choose a room with adequate space for physical exam maneuvers and allows patient to sit, lay down, and stand [3].
    - Patient should wear comfortable clothing: loose clothing such as shorts, T-shirts, tank tops to allow patient to perform appropriate physical exam maneuvers [3].
    - May ask for the assistance of another person to manage camera angles or set up camera to be able to easily adjust angles [3].
- At the start of the appointment, confirm the patient's identity and obtain consent to move forward with the telemedicine visit. Then, give patient a brief overview of what the telemedicine visit will encompass [1].
- Conduct the telemedicine visit as you would a normal visit. Start with chief complaint, history of present illness or interim

history, review of systems, then move on to physical exam maneuvers [1]:
- Inspection/observation through the camera—asymmetry, edema, discoloration/erythema, bony or soft tissue deformities.
- Palpation—patient will perform. Locate any areas of tenderness, increased warmth, crepitus.
- Range of motion—model movements for patient.
- Neurologic examination:
    Muscle strength testing—can use household objects or another person to test resistance.
    Sensation—can use cotton swab for light tough, safety pin for pinprick.
- Reflex testing—can be done by another person with side of hand or object with flat side.
- Special tests.
- Gait if applicable.
- After history and physical, give assessment and plan.
- Ask patient if he/she has any questions.
- Set up follow-up.

References

1. Verduzco-Gutierrez M, Bean AC, Tenforde AS, Tapia RN, Silver JK. How to conduct an outpatient telemedicine rehabilitation or prehabilitation visit. J Injury Funct Rehabil. 2020;12:714–20. https://doi.org/10.1002/pmrj.12380.
2. Whitney S, Atala A, Terlecki R, Kelly E, Matthews C. Implementation guide for rapid integration of an outpatient telemedicine program during the COVID-19 pandemic. J Am Coll Surg. 2020;2:216–22. https://doi.org/10.1016/j.jamcollsurg.2020.04.030.
3. Laskowski ER, Johnson SE, Shelerud RA, Lee JA, Rabatin AE, Driscoll SW, Moore BJ, Wainberg MC, Terzic CM. The telemedicine musculoskeletal examination. Mayo Clin Proc. 2020;95(8):1715–31. https://doi.org/10.1016/j.mayocp.2020.05.026.

The General Telemedicine Exam

3

Elinor H. Naor

Chief Complaint/Patient History

The physical exam should be focused based on the patient's chief complaint and reported history. Physical exam intuition and confidence gained with experience may be muted when adapting to the televisit format. This is why practitioners need to make the most of their auditory and visual skills. While in the standard musculoskeletal patient the general physical exam may seem of low importance compared to a focused exam of the extremity involved; the general exam can reveal underlying systemic medical issues which could be missed on a focused assessment alone.

When obtaining a history, it is important to note signs of systemic disease. Patients should be asked about recent weight loss (associated with malignancy), fatigue (associated with autoimmune disease), skin changes (associated with autoimmune disease), fevers (associated with infectious etiologies, and family history (associated with genetic factors). In addition, the location and onset of pain can point to specific causes of disease. Note in a patient complaining of joint pain, if it is polyarticular versus monoarticular; are the joints involved symmetric or asymmetric.

E. H. Naor (✉)
Department of Physical Medicine and Rehabilitation, Mount Sinai Hospital, New York, NY, USA
e-mail: elinor.naor@mountsinai.org

© The Author(s), under exclusive license to Springer Nature Switzerland AG 2023
M. Zakhary et al. (eds.), *Telemedicine for the Musculoskeletal Physical Exam*, https://doi.org/10.1007/978-3-031-16873-4_3

If a patient is presenting with muscle weakness—identify if the affected muscle groups are proximal versus peripheral.

The recommendations made for the treatment of musculoskeletal disorders should take into consideration pulmonary, cardiac, gastrointestinal, and genitourinary issues. These systems are not the primary focus of the musculoskeletal exam so should only be thoroughly assessed when appropriate.

Physical Exam

Initial Setup (Suggestions on how to visually optimize)

Initially ask the patient to place themselves in the direct view of the camera. Ideally, the patient should be visualized from their head down to the waist. The skin should be exposed at the level that is comfortable for the patient; men should expose their full chest and women wear a sports bra or tank-top.

Inspection/Observation

General

A patient's general appearance is noted in the first moments of every encounter. Practitioners should pay close attention not only to the patient's appearance, but also to the pace and content of their speech. Physicians should note a patient's mood and behavior; do they appear their stated age? Are they well kept or disheveled? Assumptions can be made based on these observations about socioeconomic status, fitness level, and nutrition. However, they should be corroborated by questions asked and answered when obtaining a full history.

Pulmonary

Patients presenting for musculoskeletal evaluation may be unlikely to suffer active respiratory issues; however respiratory disease can interfere with exercise capacity or may be a sign of systemic disease. Providers should observe for any asymmetries in chest rise and fall, signs of respiratory distress (tachypnea, intercostal retractions, pursed lips, accessory muscle use), signs of cyanosis (proximal or peripheral), clubbing of the fingers, and respiratory rate (a normal respiratory rate is between 13 and 20 bpm). If there is access to virtually compatible auscultatory devices, patients can be instructed on anterior or lateral chest placement—if someone else is present they can place said device as well. Examples of noteworthy auscultatory findings are wheezing and stridor. Wheezing is described as a high-pitched breath sound. Expiratory wheeze is associated with asthma. Stridor is an inspiratory wheeze that can be heard loudest in the neck is associated with upper airway obstruction. Pulmonary exam is discussed in detail in Chap. 14.

Cardiovascular

If possible, observe the patient's exposed chest. Identify any surgical scars, or evidence of a pacemaker in place. The ideal position to examine a patient for cardiac pathology is with the patient supine with the head of the bed elevated to 30°. This position can be difficult to produce during a televisit. If possible, direct the camera to the neck to assess jugular venous pulsations. In addition, limbs should be examined for splinter hemorrhages, Osler's nodes, Janeway lesions, tendon xanthomas, vascular skin changes, or dependent/pitting edema. Normal heart sounds are described as S1 and S2 and are auscultated at the right second intercostal space lateral to the sternum (aortic area), at the left second intercostal space lateral to the sternum (pulmonary area), at the left fourth intercostal space lateral to the sternum (tricuspid area), and at the left fifth intercostal space midclavicular line (mitral area). If an S4 heart sound is present, this may be a sign of heart failure. Practitioners should note heart sound intensity, location, and when they occur in the cardiac cycle. They should note any abnormalities and irregularities in rate, rhythm, and if murmurs are present.

Gastrointestinal

Initially, assess the patient's skin and eyes for evidence of jaundice. Observe the abdomen for asymmetry or masses. Note if there is evidence of abdominal distention, scars, hyperpigmentation, Cullen's sign, Grey-Turner sign, ecchymosis, or striae. The abdomen may be auscultated as well using a virtually compatible stethoscope. Make sure to instruct the patient to auscultate before palpation as it may influence bowel sounds. Normal bowel sounds consist of gurgles at a rate of 5–30 per minute. An occasional loud sustained gurgle may be heard as well. If no bowel sounds are heard over a minute, this may be a sign of constipation. If bowel sounds are heard more frequently than 30 per min, this is a sign of hyperactive bowel noted when the patient has recently eaten or is experiencing diarrhea.

Genitourinary

Given the sensitivity of doing a genitourinary exam providers should be cautious when deciding to examine this organ system in the telehealth setting. Patients should be reassured that a secure channel is used for the telehealth visit and providers must be sensitive to their comfort level. Providers should ascertain if patients are experiencing saddle paresthesia, urinary incontinence, urinary frequency, or urinary retention. These could be warning signs of nerve compression that must be addressed emergently.

Palpation

Pulmonary

If the patient is reporting pain with breathing, it is important to assess if this pain is reproducible on exam by asking them to apply pressure to the site of pain. For more details on the pulmonary exam, refer to Chap. 14.

Cardiovascular

Patients who do not own a pulse oximeter or smartwatch with similar capabilities, should be instructed on how to check their own pulse. A simple instruction can be for example: "Trace your index and middle finger pads down the inside of the thumb until you reach the wrist at a point between the bone and the tendon. Apply light pressure and feel for a pulse. You can either count the beats yourself or let me assess it by saying 'now' every time you feel a pulse." This technique can also be used when assessing pedal pulses.

Gastrointestinal
If a patient is complaining of abdominal tenderness, it can be difficult to ask said patient to palpate their abdomen. Patients should be asked to apply pressure in all nine quadrants of their abdomen and report if they feel masses or pain. To perform percussion and special tests of the gastrointestinal system properly, a medical provider must be present in person and therefore it will not be discussed in detail—this is true of the genitourinary system as well.

Genitourinary System
Similarly to the abdominal exam, the patient can be instructed to palpate their suprapubic region for masses or tenderness. Providers should ascertain if the patient is experiencing saddle anesthesia both from the history and by the patients palpating on the groin/pubic region on their own.

Differential Diagnosis

Once a proper history and physical is obtained, a list of differential diagnoses can be compiled. If patients are showing signs of pulmonary pathologies in the form of cyanosis or abnormal pattern of breathing; vagus nerve injury, COPD, or asthma should be considered. Cardiovascular pathologies are vast and numerous and physicians should know the symptoms of diseases such as heart failure and intermittent claudication so that referrals are placed in a timely manner. Signs of bowel and bladder incontinence, retention, or constipation can be signs of severe pathology such as spinal cord injury or as mild as a medication side effect (opiates, anticholinergics). Below we will discuss examples of disease processes that have musculoskeletal, as well as non-musculoskeletal manifestations. In these cases, the general exam may play an important role in diagnosis and subsequent management.

Marfan Syndrome

Marfan syndrome is a hereditary systemic tissue disorder that is most commonly a result of a mutation in the Fibrillin 1 gene. Systemic signs may include ectopic lens, wrist/thumb sign, pectus carinatum, hindfoot valgus, pneumothorax, dural ectasia, protrusio acetabuli, mitral valve prolapse, myopia, scoliosis, increase arm span, reduced elbow extension, or skin striae. Aortic findings in patients with Marfan syndrome under 20 years old is a diameter greater than 3 cm and in those under 20 years old is greater than 2 cm. In addition, they are at high risk of aortic root dissection. Of note, patients will likely have excess length of long bones and increased joint laxity. To be diagnosed with Marfan syndrome, the following criteria must be met:

1. If they do not have a family history of Marfan syndrome, but do have an aortic diameter equal to or greater than two as well as systemic symptoms, or fibrillin gene mutation.
2. If they do have a family history of Marfan syndrome and systemic symptoms [1].

Dermatomyositis/Polymyositis

Dermatomyositis (DM) and polymyositis (PM) are idiopathic inflammatory myopathies that present with proximal muscle weakness due to inflammation. Dermatomyositis is identified based on its cutaneous manifestation, which includes Gottron papules and heliotrope rash. On lab analysis patients will have elevated inflammatory markers. Diagnosis of PM and DM is made with muscle biopsy; displaying muscle fiber necrosis, degeneration, regeneration with the presence of inflammatory cells [2].

Systemic Lupus Erythematosus

Systemic lupus erythematosus (SLE) is a chronic autoimmune disease with numerous clinical manifestations. Patients may present with systemic symptoms such as fatigue, fever, or weight loss.

The musculoskeletal manifestations include symmetrical migratory polyarthropathy resolving within 24 h primarily affecting the joints of the knees, and proximal interphalangeal joints. On physical exam, some patients will have flexion, deformity, ulnar deviation of the wrist, swan neck deformity, Raynaud's phenomenon, or tendinitis [3, 4]. The diagnosis of SLE is described by the SLICC 2019 criteria or The European League Against Rheumatism (EULAR)/American College of Rheumatology (ACR) classification criteria for SLE [5]. A diagnosis of SLE is confirmed in patients that have a positive ANA in addition to a scoring system based on seven clinical and three immunologic signs; a score of 10 confirms the diagnosis.

Spondyloarthropathies

Spondyloarthropathies are a group of diseased who share a set of clinical characteristics. Patients typically present with back pain, asymmetric oligoarthritis affecting the lower extremity, enthesis, and dactylitis. Symptom onset is typically in the 40th decade of life. Back pain is typically acute, worse at night, and improves with exercise [6]. Imaging usually shows axial joint inflammation affecting the SI joint most commonly (sacroiliitis) and labs will have elevated inflammatory markers and are positive for HLA B27 [7]. The diseases that fall within this category are: ankylosing spondylitis, reactive arthritis, juvenile onset spondyloarthropathy, spondyloarthropathy associated with IBD, spondyloarthropathy associated with psoriasis, peripheral spondyloarthropathy, and non-radiographic axial spondyloarthropathy [8]. Non-musculoskeletal manifestation will involve the eyes (conjunctivitis, uveitis), skin, immune, and GI system. The diagnosis of the spondyloarthropathies is made based on axial and peripheral manifestations.

1. Axial: History of idiopathic back pain manifesting itself before the age of 45 lasting for at least 3 months. Criteria: either HLA-B27 positive or sacroiliitis on imaging as well as one-two additional features (inflammatory back pain, arthritis, heel enthesitis, uveitis, psoriasis, IBD, dactylitis, elevated inflammatory markers, family history of spondyloarthropathy) [9].

2. Peripheral: Patients with symptoms of arthritis, enthesis, and dactylitis as well as one group A feature and two group B features.
   (a) Group A: Uveitis, psoriasis, IBD, history of genitourinary infection, HLA-B27 positive, sacroiliitis.
   (b) Group B: Arthritis, enthesis, dactylitis, history of inflammatory back pain, family history of spondyloarthropathy [10].

Rheumatic Fever

Rheumatic fever is a clinical sequelae of group A streptococcal (GAS) pharyngitis that presents 1–5 weeks after initial infection. Clinical manifestations include: arthritis, pancarditis, subcutaneous nodules, chorea, and erythema marginatum. The most common cardiac pathology is endocarditis of the mitral or aortic valve causing regurgitation. Mitral valve regurgitation (MVR) will be heard on cardiac exam as a pansystolic murmur best heard at the apex. Aortic regurgitation (AR) is heard on exam as an end diastolic murmur that is loudest at the right second intercostal space. If the valvular dysfunction is severe, it may result in heart failure. The (Sydenham) chorea typically presents as weakness, emotional disturbance, and acute unilateral interrupted movements that worsen with intention [11]. The erythema marginatum lesions are non-pruritic, worse in heat, and come and go [12]. Patients present with transient ascending migratory polyarthritis [11]. The subcutaneous nodules are painless and found on the extensor surfaces. The diagnosis of rheumatic fever is made using the Jones Criteria. Diagnosis is divided into two types: initial episode, and recurrent.

1. An initial episode in patients with a history of GAS infection presents with two major features or one major and two minor features.
2. A recurrent episode will present with two major, one major and two minor, or three minor.
   (a) Major criteria: Carditis, arthritis chorea, erythema marginatum, and subcutaneous nodules.

3. Minor criteria: Polyarthralgia, fever sedimentation rate ≥60 mm and/or C-reactive protein ≥3.0 mg/dL, and prolonged PR interval.

Management/Treatment

Marfan Syndrome

The management of Marfan syndrome is multifactorial but most importantly includes monitoring of the diameter of the aortic root. Patients at risk of aortic aneurysm benefit from a long-acting beta-blocker or ACE inhibitor. Ocular pathologies may be treated with vision correction and photocoagulation. Mitral valve repair is indicated in patients with severe MVR. If scoliosis is present, depending on its severity; exercise, bracing, and therapy are beneficial. If the scoliosis is severe (COB angle >40), spinal fusion should be considered. In terms of exercise intensity and restriction, the American Heart Association has made the following recommendations for patients with Marfan syndrome:

1. Low to moderate intensity exercise such as jogging, swimming, or bowling is likely permissible.
2. If cleared by a cardiologist, may participate in intermediate intensity exercise.
3. Patients may not participate in contact spots, high intensity exercise, isometric exercise that may produce a Valsalva maneuver.
4. Patients shouldn't engage in scuba diving due to the risk of pneumothorax secondary to barotrauma [13].

Dermatomyositis/Polymyositis

Patients with DM/PM benefit from pharmacologic therapies. It has been found that steroid therapy preserves muscle function and improves strength and is typically tapered over a year [14]. Usually, 3 months after initiating pharmacotherapy, patients will achieve maximal muscle recovery [14]. If steroids are ineffective or contraindicated, azathioprine and methotrexate are recommended treatments as well. In severe cases, presenting with dysphagia and risk of aspiration both glucocorticoids and intravenous immunoglobulin are indicated [15]. Of note, involvement of the cricopharyngeal muscle increases risk of aspiration; in this situation, a referral to speech therapy is essential.

In terms of exercise tolerance and benefit, there isn't sufficient evidence-based medicine in support or against this approach. Passive range of motion has been found to be helpful in patients with severe weakness. In addition, steps should be taken to prevent contractures such as bracing and stretching. Patients who have regained a muscle strength of four or greater may participate in isometric and resistive exercises. If able, patients should be instructed on home exercises and encouraged to participate in vigorous isotonic exercises [16].

Systemic Lupus Erythematosus

SLE treatment varies depending on clinical manifestations of the flare up and patients' response. For systemic symptoms hydroxychloroquine, nonsteroidal anti-inflammatory (NSAIDs), glucocorticosteroids (short course: 2–4 weeks) are first line. If patients experience symptoms refractory to first line medications, disease-modifying antirheumatic drugs (DMARDs) are recommended [17]. Those who still don't experience relief with a 3-to-6-month course of methotrexate/leflunomide can try azathioprine—if this too is ineffective, belimumab should be started [18–20]. Studies have shown that patients with symptoms of muscle weakness and fatigue benefit from graded aerobic exercise programs [21].

Spondyloarthropathies

Patients diagnosed with any of the spondyloarthropathies should be referred to appropriate specialists, determined by their presenting symptoms. Specialists may include rheumatologist, dermatologist, gastroenterologist, and ophthalmologist. Pharmacologic treatment is variable by disease severity and includes: NSAIDs, DMARDs, biologics, and intra-articular injections. NSAIDs (naproxen, celecoxib, or ibuprofen) should be tried initially and are beneficial in most patients [22]. If after 4 weeks of NSAIDs pain has not resolved, TNF-alpha inhibitors are recommended. If TNF-alpha inhibitors are also non-beneficial, this may be an indication for DMARDs or eventually biologic agents [23]. Patients with severe peripheral arthropathy who fail a few weeks of prednisone may benefit from DMARDs therapy as well [24]. Exercise can be helpful for these patients in conjunction with medications. Physical therapists should work on postural exercise training, range of motion exercises, recreational therapy, stretching, and hydrotherapy. If symptoms are severe, patients should be referred to intense care in the setting of acute rehabilitation [22, 25].

Rheumatic Fever

The best way to treat rheumatic fever is with prevention, which in this case can be achieved with proper treatment of strep pharyngitis. Patients suffering from carditis should be referred to a cardiologist for assessment of disease severity and medication recommendations. In order to prevent recurrence of rheumatic heart disease, patients are prescribed prophylactic antibiotics [26]. Patients with symptoms of Sydenham chorea benefit from psychological and social support. This movement disorder, usually resolved on its own, however for severe symptoms carbamazepine can be used. The arthritis symptoms typically resolve within 4 weeks and don't result in long-term joint deformity [11]. For joint pain, NSAIDS can be used initially (6-to-12-week course). If pain is refractory to NSAIDs, a steroid taper is recommended. Exercise tolerance is dependent on severity of cardiac disease and a cardiologist should be consulted for clearance.

Complications/Red Flags

In the general exam, clinician should make sure to keep a lookout for red flags in their history and physical exam. When obtaining a history note oncological history, smoking history, recent weight loss, point tenderness, or localized swelling, over weeks to months. If malignancy is suspected, X-ray should be ordered as well as ESR (if <20, unlikely secondary to malignancy) [27]. If patients report new or progressively worsening neurological symptoms or are experiencing bowel and bladder incontinence, saddle paresthesia, practitioners should be concerned about possible cauda equina or cord compression. In these cases, an emergent MRI should be ordered. Patients reporting fevers, tenderness to palpation, may have an infectious cause to their musculoskeletal complaints. Those who are immunocompromised are at risk. Risk factories are being on hemodialysis or immunosuppressant, or a history of IV drug use, spinal procedures, endocarditis, and bacteremia. If an infectious source is suspected, an MRI should be ordered to rule out spinal abscess, or a radionuclide scan can be ordered to rule out osteomyelitis. Patients reporting severe pain in a single joint with evidence of swelling or erythema should be worked up for crystal-induced arthropathy (gout, pseudogout). If patients have a history of trauma, or risk factors for osteoporosis (e.g., advanced in age or prolonged steroid use) and are presenting with acute localized pain, have X-ray ordered to rule out fracture. The faster proper imaging is obtained, the sooner patients can receive appropriate and timely treatments.

References

1. Loeys BL, Dietz HC, Braverman AC, Callewaert BL, De Backer J, Devereux RB, Hilhorst-Hofstee Y, Jondeau G, Faivre L, Milewicz DM, Pyeritz RE, Sponseller PD, Wordsworth P, De Paepe AM. The revised Ghent nosology for the Marfan syndrome. J Med Genet. 2010;47(7):476–85. https://doi.org/10.1136/jmg.2009.072785.
2. Dalakas MC, Hohlfeld R. Polymyositis and dermatomyositis. Lancet. 2003;362(9388):971–82. https://doi.org/10.1016/S0140-6736(03)14368-1.

3. Cronin ME. Musculoskeletal manifestations of systemic lupus erythematosus. Rheum Dis Clin North Am. 1988;14(1):99–116.
4. Grossman JM. Lupus arthritis. Best Pract Res Clin Rheumatol. 2009;23(4):495–506. https://doi.org/10.1016/j.berh.2009.04.003.
5. Aringer M, Costenbader K, Daikh D, Brinks R, Mosca M, Ramsey-Goldman R, Smolen JS, Wofsy D, Boumpas DT, Kamen DL, Jayne D, Cervera R, Costedoat-Chalumeau N, Diamond B, Gladman DD, Hahn B, Hiepe F, Jacobsen S, Khanna D, Lerstrøm K, Massarotti E, McCune J, Ruiz-Irastorza G, Sanchez-Guerrero J, Schneider M, Urowitz M, Bertsias G, Hoyer BF, Leuchten N, Tani C, Tedeschi SK, Touma Z, Schmajuk G, Anic B, Assan F, Chan TM, Clarke AE, Crow MK, Czirják L, Doria A, Graninger W, Halda-Kiss B, Hasni S, Izmirly PM, Jung M, Kumánovics G, Mariette X, Padjen I, Pego-Reigosa JM, Romero-Diaz J, Rúa-Figueroa Fernández Í, Seror R, Stummvoll GH, Tanaka Y, Tektonidou MG, Vasconcelos C, Vital EM, Wallace DJ, Yavuz S, Meroni PL, Fritzler MJ, Naden R, Dörner T, Johnson SR. 2019 European League Against Rheumatism/American College of Rheumatology classification criteria for systemic lupus erythematosus. Ann Rheum Dis. 2019;78(9):1151–9. https://doi.org/10.1136/annrheumdis-2018-214819.
6. Rudwaleit M, van der Heijde D, Khan MA, Braun J, Sieper J. How to diagnose axial spondyloarthritis early. Ann Rheum Dis. 2004;63(5):535–43. https://doi.org/10.1136/ard.2003.011247.
7. Sepriano A, Ramiro S, van der Heijde D, van Gaalen F, Hoonhout P, Molto A, Saraux A, Ramonda R, Dougados M, Landewé R. What is axial spondyloarthritis? A latent class and transition analysis in the SPACE and DESIR cohorts (Erratum in: Ann Rheum Dis 2020;79(6):e78). Ann Rheum Dis. 2020;79(3):324–31. https://doi.org/10.1136/annrheumdis-2019-216516.
8. Zeidler H, Calin A, Amor B. A historical perspective of the spondyloarthritis. Curr Opin Rheumatol. 2011;23(4):327–33. https://doi.org/10.1097/BOR.0b013e3283470ecd.
9. Rudwaleit M, van der Heijde D, Landewé R, Listing J, Akkoc N, Brandt J, Braun J, Chou CT, Collantes-Estevez E, Dougados M, Huang F, Gu J, Khan MA, Kirazli Y, Maksymowych WP, Mielants H, Sørensen IJ, Ozgocmen S, Roussou E, Valle-Oñate R, Weber U, Wei J, Sieper J. The development of Assessment of Spondyloarthritis International Society classification criteria for axial spondyloarthritis (part II): validation and final selection (Erratum in: Ann Rheum Dis. 2019;78(6):e59.). Ann Rheum Dis. 2009;68(6):777–83. https://doi.org/10.1136/ard.2009.108233.
10. Rudwaleit M, van der Heijde D, Landewé R, Akkoc N, Brandt J, Chou CT, Dougados M, Huang F, Gu J, Kirazli Y, Van den Bosch F, Olivieri I, Roussou E, Scarpato S, Sørensen IJ, Valle-Oñate R, Weber U, Wei J, Sieper J. The assessment of SpondyloArthritis International Society classification criteria for peripheral spondyloarthritis and for spondyloarthri-

tis in general. Ann Rheum Dis. 2011;70(1):25–31. https://doi.org/10.1136/ard.2010.133645.
11. Gewitz MH, Baltimore RS, Tani LY, Sable CA, Shulman ST, Carapetis J, Remenyi B, Taubert KA, Bolger AF, Beerman L, Mayosi BM, Beaton A, Pandian NG, Kaplan EL, American Heart Association Committee on Rheumatic Fever, Endocarditis, and Kawasaki Disease of the Council on Cardiovascular Disease in the Young. Revision of the Jones Criteria for the diagnosis of acute rheumatic fever in the era of Doppler echocardiography: a scientific statement from the American Heart Association (Erratum in: Circulation. 2020 Jul 28;142(4):e65.). Circulation. 2015;131(20):1806–18.https://doi.org/10.1161/CIR.0000000000000205.
12. Feinstein AR, Spagnuolo M. The clinical patterns of acute rheumatic fever: a reappraisal. Medicine (Baltimore). 1962;41:279–305. https://doi.org/10.1097/00005792-196212000-00001.
13. Maron BJ, Chaitman BR, Ackerman MJ, Bayés de Luna A, Corrado D, Crosson JE, Deal BJ, Driscoll DJ, Estes NA 3rd, Araújo CG, Liang DH, Mitten MJ, Myerburg RJ, Pelliccia A, Thompson PD, Towbin JA, Van Camp SP, Working Groups of the American Heart Association Committee on Exercise, Cardiac Rehabilitation, and Prevention; Councils on Clinical Cardiology and Cardiovascular Disease in the Young. Recommendations for physical activity and recreational sports participation for young patients with genetic cardiovascular diseases. Circulation. 2004;109(22):2807–16. https://doi.org/10.1161/01.CIR.0000128363.85581.E1.
14. Drake LA, Dinehart SM, Farmer ER, Goltz RW, Graham GF, Hordinsky MK, Lewis CW, Pariser DM, Skouge JW, Webster SB, Whitaker DC, Butler B, Lowery BJ, Sontheimer RD, Callen JP, Camisa C, Provost TT, Tuffanelli DL. Guidelines of care for dermatomyositis. American Academy of Dermatology. J Am Acad Dermatol. 1996;34(5 Pt 1):824–9.
15. Marie I, Menard JF, Hatron PY, Hachulla E, Mouthon L, Tiev K, Ducrotte P, Cherin P. Intravenous immunoglobulins for steroid-refractory esophageal involvement related to polymyositis and dermatomyositis: a series of 73 patients. Arthritis Care Res (Hoboken). 2010;62(12):1748–55. https://doi.org/10.1002/acr.20325.
16. Dastmalchi M, Alexanderson H, Loell I, Ståhlberg M, Borg K, Lundberg IE, Esbjörnsson M. Effect of physical training on the proportion of slow-twitch type I muscle fibers, a novel nonimmune-mediated mechanism for muscle impairment in polymyositis or dermatomyositis. Arthritis Rheum. 2007;57(7):1303–10. https://doi.org/10.1002/art.22996.
17. Williams HJ, Egger MJ, Singer JZ, Willkens RF, Kalunian KC, Clegg DO, Skosey JL, Brooks RH, Alarcón GS, Steen VD, et al. Comparison of hydroxychloroquine and placebo in the treatment of the arthropathy of mild systemic lupus erythematosus. J Rheumatol. 1994;21(8):1457–62.
18. Remer CF, Weisman MH, Wallace DJ. Benefits of leflunomide in systemic lupus erythematosus: a pilot observational study. Lupus. 2001;10(7):480–3. https://doi.org/10.1191/096120301678416033.

19. Hahn BH, Kantor OS, Osterland CK. Azathioprine plus prednisone compared with prednisone alone in the treatment of systemic lupus erythematosus. Report of a prospective controlled trial in 24 patients. Ann Intern Med. 1975;83(5):597–605. https://doi.org/10.7326/0003-4819-83-5-597.
20. Furie R, Petri M, Zamani O, Cervera R, Wallace DJ, Tegzová D, Sanchez-Guerrero J, Schwarting A, Merrill JT, Chatham WW, Stohl W, Ginzler EM, Hough DR, Zhong ZJ, Freimuth W, van Vollenhoven RF, BLISS-76 Study Group. A phase III, randomized, placebo-controlled study of belimumab, a monoclonal antibody that inhibits B lymphocyte stimulator, in patients with systemic lupus erythematosus. Arthritis Rheum. 2011;63(12):3918–30. https://doi.org/10.1002/art.30613.
21. Tench CM, McCarthy J, McCurdie I, White PD, D'Cruz DP. Fatigue in systemic lupus erythematosus: a randomized controlled trial of exercise. Rheumatology (Oxford). 2003;42(9):1050–4. https://doi.org/10.1093/rheumatology/keg289.
22. Dagfinrud H, Kvien TK, Hagen KB. Physiotherapy interventions for ankylosing spondylitis. Cochrane Database Syst Rev. 2008;1:CD002822. https://doi.org/10.1002/14651858.CD002822.pub3.
23. Ward MM, Deodhar A, Gensler LS, Dubreuil M, Yu D, Khan MA, Haroon N, Borenstein D, Wang R, Biehl A, Fang MA, Louie G, Majithia V, Ng B, Bigham R, Pianin M, Shah AA, Sullivan N, Turgunbaev M, Oristaglio J, Turner A, Maksymowych WP, Caplan L. 2019 Update of the American College of Rheumatology/Spondylitis Association of America/Spondyloarthritis Research and Treatment Network recommendations for the treatment of ankylosing spondylitis and nonradiographic axial spondyloarthritis. Arthritis Rheumatol. 2019;71(10):1599–613. https://doi.org/10.1002/art.41042.
24. Ward MM, Deodhar A, Gensler LS, Dubreuil M, Yu D, Khan MA, Haroon N, Borenstein D, Wang R, Biehl A, Fang MA, Louie G, Majithia V, Ng B, Bigham R, Pianin M, Shah AA, Sullivan N, Turgunbaev M, Oristaglio J, Turner A, Maksymowych WP, Caplan L. 2019 Update of the American College of Rheumatology/Spondylitis Association of America/Spondyloarthritis Research and Treatment Network recommendations for the treatment of ankylosing spondylitis and nonradiographic axial spondyloarthritis. Arthritis Care Res (Hoboken). 2019;71(10):1285–99. https://doi.org/10.1002/acr.24025.
25. Lubrano E, D'Angelo S, Parsons WJ, Corbi G, Ferrara N, Rengo F, Olivieri I. Effectiveness of rehabilitation in active ankylosing spondylitis assessed by the ASAS response criteria. Rheumatology (Oxford). 2007;46(11):1672–5. https://doi.org/10.1093/rheumatology/kem247.
26. Gerber MA, Baltimore RS, Eaton CB, Gewitz M, Rowley AH, Shulman ST, Taubert KA. Prevention of rheumatic fever and diagnosis and treatment of acute streptococcal pharyngitis: a scientific statement from the American Heart Association Rheumatic Fever, Endocarditis, and Kawasaki Disease Committee of the Council on Cardiovascular Disease

in the young, the interdisciplinary council on functional genomics and translational biology, and the interdisciplinary council on quality of care and outcomes research: endorsed by the American Academy of Pediatrics. Circulation. 2009;119(11):1541–51. https://doi.org/10.1161/CIRCULATIONAHA.109.191959.

27. Deyo RA, Diehl AK. Cancer as a cause of back pain: frequency, clinical presentation, and diagnostic strategies. J Gen Intern Med. 1988;3(3):230–8. https://doi.org/10.1007/BF02596337.

The Telemedicine Cervical Spine Exam

4

Chandni Patel, Jonathan Ramin, and David A. Spinner

Telemedicine is the practice of remotely providing patient care through the application of a technology. The availability of modern technology, specifically the use of a camera and live video conferencing, has facilitated telemedicine and transformed the way clinicians can treat patients. Clinicians will rely greatly on patient history and participation in physical examination in evaluating etiology of symptoms. This chapter will discuss the approach to a cervical spine musculoskeletal exam via telemedicine.

Chief Complaint/Patient History

For the cervical spine, patients may present to a telemedicine visit with a myriad of complaints including headaches, neck pain, upper extremity pain, upper extremity paresthesias, and/or upper extremity weakness. A detailed history should be obtained to help narrow down where the symptoms are likely derived from. Patients may not associate certain upper motor neuron signs as coming from the neck, and hence it is vital to include such

C. Patel (✉) · J. Ramin · D. A. Spinner
Department of Rehabilitation and Human Performance, Icahn School of Medicine at Mount Sinai, New York, NY, USA
e-mail: chandni.patel@mountsinai.org; jonathan.ramin@mountsinai.org; david.spinner@mountsinai.org

© The Author(s), under exclusive license to Springer Nature Switzerland AG 2023
M. Zakhary et al. (eds.), *Telemedicine for the Musculoskeletal Physical Exam*, https://doi.org/10.1007/978-3-031-16873-4_4

questions in your history. This includes questions about difficulties with balance, bowel or bladder incontinence, and/or saddle anesthesia. For this reason, a thorough history and examination of joints above and below the suspected source of pain should be examined. For the cervical spine, this should include the shoulder and in some instances a thorough neurologic examination including cranial nerves, mental status, coordination, and gait.

Physical Exam

Initiation of a successful telemedicine visit begins with proper setup of the patient and surrounding environment. First, ensure proper lighting is available to evaluate the patient. Next, make certain there is adequate space surrounding the patient to perform the physical examination. Ensure the patient is wearing proper clothing revealing the cervical spine, upper thoracic spine, and shoulders. The camera should then be adjusted to adequately visualize the area of concern. Ultimately, there should be privacy for both the examiner and patient with minimal distractions. The examiner's surrounding environment should also be set up similarly to the patient so that they may be able to demonstrate portions of the exam for patients when necessary.

Inspection

After establishing an optimal environment, the musculoskeletal cervical spine physical examination will begin with inspection. Have the patient stand in front of the camera with feet shoulder width apart, forward facing, and arms to the side. From the anterior view, evaluate for head tilt, facial asymmetry, clavicular and shoulder levelness, elbow rotation carrying angle, patella heights, valgus or varus deformities of the hips or knees, and for any pronation or supination of feet [1].

Then have the patient turn 90° to the right or left of the screen to provide a lateral postural view. Evaluate the position of the head in relation to the line of gravity which passes through the external auditory meatus, the acromioclavicular joint, the greater trochanter, and anterior to lateral malleolus [1]. Specifically, evaluate for head posture, cervical, thoracic, and lumbar curvatures lordosis, rounded shoulders or flexion or hyperextension of the knees.

For the last view of postural assessment, have the patient turn an additional 90° to facilitate examination in the posterior view. In this view, evaluate for side bending or rotation of the head, mastoid process, shoulder levelness, inferior tips of the scapula, gluteal crease level, popliteal line levels, and aches of the feet [1].

It is important to examine the overlying skin and muscle bulk when examining the patient in the anterior, lateral, and posterior views for changes in overlying skin, rashes, erythema, or ecchymosis. Additionally, evaluation of asymmetry in skin or muscles should be examined for atrophy or underlying effusions.

Palpation

An important part of musculoskeletal examination is palpation. With examination over telemedicine, the patient should be instructed to palpate for areas of tenderness with one finger. Specifically, guide the patient over the spinous processes of the cervical spine, occiput, cervical and upper thoracic paraspinal muscles, trapezius, levator scapulae, and sternocleidomastoid muscles. Areas of tenderness can be further examined by instructing the patient to press deeper for a deeper examination.

Range of Motion

Movement at the cervical spine can be assessed by having the patient move through active ranges of motion in flexion, extension, lateral bending, and rotation. To begin, have the patient sit or stand in front of the camera. Instruct the patient to bring his or her chin to chest to evaluate flexion of the cervical spine. Then have the patient move their head back into extension by looking up towards the ceiling.

Next, have the patient rotate their head to the left and right while the examiner compares each side to decipher any asymmetries in motion. Finally, have the patient laterally bend the neck by bringing each ear to its corresponding shoulder. While evaluating the range of motion of the cervical spine, take note of any movements that either trigger or alleviate their symptoms and the location of the pain.

Additionally, range of motion of the shoulder should be evaluated for possible pain reproduction or alternative sources of pain. Refer to "The Musculoskeletal Shoulder Exam" chapter for a guide on proper evaluation of the shoulder.

Neurological Examination

Muscle Strength Testing

Muscle strength can be tested using common household items of known weights. The object should be able to fit in the hand of the patient. Each spinal nerve root level can be tested from C5–T1. Using the object and lifting against gravity, the following muscles should be tested:

(a) The deltoid should be tested with shoulder abduction, testing the C5/C6 nerve root and axillary nerve.
(b) The biceps should be tested with elbow flexion, testing the C5/C6 (predominantly C5) nerve roots and musculocutaneous nerve.
(c) The extensor carpi radialis should be tested with wrist extension, testing the C6/C7 (predominantly C6) nerve root and radial nerve.
(d) The triceps should be tested with elbow extension, testing the C5/C6/C7 (predominantly C7) nerve root and radial nerve.
(e) The abductor digiti minimi should be tested with finger abduction, testing the C8/T1 (predominantly C8) nerve root and ulnar nerve.
(f) The flexor digitorum profundus should be tested with distal interphalangeal joint flexion of the middle finger, testing the C8/T1 (predominantly T1) nerve root and median nerve.

If the patient is able to move the joint through full range of motion with the weight, then a muscle grade of at least 4/5 may be given for that specific myotome.

Sensation

Initial sensation testing can begin by asking the patient to identify any areas of abnormal sensation. Specifically have the patient outline this region with their finger. Sensation testing can be further broken down by testing light touch, pinprick, temperature, and vibration. Start by demonstrating the method on yourself to the patient. Light touch can be tested by having the patient use a cotton swab to examine specific skin areas. For pin prick testing, have patients unfold a paperclip or use a toothpick. Using the tools of choice, the following dermatomes should be tested:

(a) C2: 1 centimeter lateral to the occipital protuberance
(b) C3: supraclavicular fossa
(c) C4: tip of acromion
(d) C5: lateral epicondyle
(e) C6: thumb
(f) C7: middle finger
(g) C8: fifth digit
(h) T1: medial epicondyle

Reflexes

Reflexes are an important part of the physical examination in patients presenting with cervical complaints although it can be challenging to test reflexes via telemedicine. While demonstrating, have the patient use the edge of his smartphone to elicit the following reflexes.

(a) **C5**/C6: biceps
(b) C5/**C6**: brachioradialis
(c) C6/C7: pronator teres
(d) **C7**/C8: triceps

Special Tests

Spurling's Neck Compression Test

Spurling's neck compression is used to test for cervical nerve root irritation and radiculopathy. To perform the Spurling's neck compression test, have the patient seated. Begin by having the patient extend their neck back fully and rotate to the affected side. While in this position, have either the patient or an assistant (i.e., a family member or friend whom the patient is comfortable including in the telemedicine visit) apply downward pressure on their head providing a compressive force through the cervical spine. A test is considered to be positive if there is radicular pain or paresthesias into the upper extremity of the side in which the head is rotated [2, 3].

L'hermitte's Test

L'hermitte's sign is generally seen in upper cervical spinal cord pathologies involving the dorsal column and may indicate pathologies such as multiple sclerosis, cervical spinal cord tumors, Behcet's syndrome, and transverse myelitis. To perform the L'hermitte's test, begin with the patient seated. Typically in an office or inpatient setting, a physician would passively flex the head forward into full flexion; however, in the telemedicine setting, a family member or friend can forward flex the patient's head. If another person is not available, the patient may actively flex their own head forward. A positive test occurs when the patient experiences an "electric" sensation down the spine or into the extremities [4].

Shoulder Abduction Test

The shoulder abduction test is used to aid in the diagnosis of cervical nerve root irritation and radiculopathy. The test may be performed seated or supine. The patient is instructed to actively abduct the ipsilateral hand and rest it on top of his head. A positive test is indicated by relief of ipsilateral cervical radicular symptoms [3].

Examination of Related Areas

Examination of the shoulder should be done with all patients presenting with cervical spine complaints. Refer to "The Musculoskeletal Shoulder Exam" chapter for a guide on navigating the musculoskeletal exam for the shoulder.

A thorough neurologic exam should be performed in patients who present with headaches and other upper motor signs that may not be directly associated with the cervical spine.

Considerations for Certain Populations

Children

In children presenting with cervical symptoms, it is important to evaluate for the presence of any red flags. In particular, cervical pain with fevers, stiff neck, or headaches should be immediately worked up for meningitis. Additionally, presence of rashes or swelling would prompt an in-person evaluation or emergency room visit on a case-to-case basis.

Rheumatoid Arthritis

Special consideration should be taken in evaluating patients with rheumatoid arthritis (RA) as it often involves the cervical spine. Specifically, RA can cause atlantoaxial joint instability by loosening ligaments surrounding the joint which can subsequently compress the spinal cord. These patients may be neurologically intact; however, important consideration should be taken in obtaining appropriate imaging and in-person follow-up [5].

Down Syndrome

As in patients with RA, children or adults with Down syndrome are at increased risk of having atlantoaxial instability which may lead to spinal cord compression [6]. Oftentimes, the diagnosis of cervical instability resulting from AA joint involvement will require imaging.

Differential Diagnosis

1. Cervical spondylosis.
   (a) Cervical radiculopathy with or without myelopathy.
      - Cervical disc herniation.
      - Cervical stenosis.
   (b) Cervical Facet syndrome.

2. Cervical sprains and strains.
3. Cervical myofascial pain.
4. Cervical spine fracture (traumatic or atraumatic).
5. Meningitis.

Management/Treatment

When implementing a treatment plan via telemedicine, it is imperative that organized and proper communication is made between the examiner, patient, and office staff. The patient should be provided with an after-visit summary which includes any new medications that were started, radiology requisitions, referrals, miscellaneous information (reading material about their diagnosis, home exercises, etc.) and follow-up instructions. Both the provider and office staff should go over the plan with the patient, leaving ample time for the patient to ask any questions they may have. Ensure the correct contact information is on file and that the patient receives all paperwork necessary before the end of the visit.

If there is a need for the patient to be evaluated by the clinician in person, that appointment should be made immediately in order to ensure patient safety and understanding of the need for closer evaluation.

Complications/Red Flags

In the telemedicine setting, evaluation for red flags is vital. The presence of red flags should prompt immediate follow-up. Specific red flags to screen for in the cervical spine for patients with neck pain include cervical myelopathy, instability, and fractures.

Cervical myelopathy can require emergent intervention. Severe progression of symptoms or loss of function in gait, balance, manual dexterity, or bowel or bladder function can be indicative of severe spinal cord compromise and should be emergently evaluated [7].

Cervical spine instability should be considered in patients with a history of trauma or significant past medical history of rheumatoid arthritis and Down syndrome.

Clinicians should be highly suspicious of cervical spine fractures in patients reporting neck pain with a history of trauma or fall. Using the Canadian C-Spine rule, imaging should be highly considered in patients aged 65 or older, dangerous mechanisms of injury, or paresthesias in the extremities [8].

Follow-Up

Follow-up appointments should be scheduled in person for patients with new findings on physical examination. As discussed above, patients with complications or red flags should follow-up in the emergency room urgently.

References

1. Seffinger MA, Hruby RJ. Chapter 3—Manual diagnostic procedures overview. Philadelphia: W.B. Saunders; 2007. p. 35–58. https://doi.org/10.1016/B978-1-4160-2384-5.50007-9.
2. Anekstein Y, Blecher R, Smorgick Y, Mirovsky Y. What is the best way to apply the Spurling test for cervical radiculopathy? Clin Orthop Relat Res. 2012;470(9):2566–72. https://doi.org/10.1007/s11999-012-2492-3.
3. Agarwal AK, Sabat S. The cervical spine. 2nd ed. Amsterdam: Elsevier; 2020. https://doi.org/10.1007/978-3-030-22173-7_52.
4. Khare S, Seth D. Lhermitte's Sign: the current status. Ann Indian Acad Neurol. 2015;18(2):154–6.
5. Gillick J, Wainwright J. Rheumatoid arthritis and the cervical spine: a review on the role of surgery. Int J Rheumatol. 2015;2015:252456.
6. Ali F, Al-Bustan M. Cervical spine abnormalities associated with Down syndrome. Int Orthop. 2006;30(4):284–9.
7. Donnally C, Hanna A. Lumbar degenerative disk disease. Treasure Island (FL): StatPearls Publishing; 2020.
8. Stiell IG, Wells GA, Vandemheen C. The Canadian C-spine rule for radiography in alert and stable trauma patients. JAMA. 2001;286(15):1841–8.

The Telemedicine Thoracic Spine Exam

David A. Spinner, Caroline Alyse Varlotta, and Alexandra Laurent

Chief Complaint/Patient History

The primary goals of the clinical assessment are to triage the chief complaint, evaluate the symptoms and signs, establish a cause, and realize the impact of the complaint on the patient's quality of life. The physician should inquire about the symptoms, characteristics of the symptoms (localization, timing, quality), impact of symptoms, alleviating or provoking factors, and any associated symptoms. The patient should use one finger to point to the area of maximal pain and delineate any radiating pain.

The dermatomes are important when a patient describes paresthesia or other sensory symptoms. Deficits in T1 would result in ADM/interossei muscle weakness, no reflex abnormalities, and medial arm sensory deficits. T2 and T4 deficits will result in no muscle weakness or reflex abnormalities, but there will be a band-like presentation based on segmental innervation. The level of the

D. A. Spinner
Department of Rehabilitation and Human Performance, Mount Sinai Hospital, New York, NY, USA
e-mail: david.spinner@mountsinai.org

C. A. Varlotta (✉) · A. Laurent
Department of Rehabilitation and Human Performance, Mount Sinai Hospital, Scarsdale, NY, USA

apex of the axilla is at T2, while the nipple line is at T4. The xiphoid process is T6, umbilicus T10, and the inguinal ligament T12.

Any history of instrumentation is important. Long fusions are especially important because longer fusions that have an upper instrumented vertebra in the upper lumbar vertebrae (L1, L2) may lead to an extremely stressed thoracolumbar junction. The pathology that results, such as pseudoarthrosis or proximal junctional kyphosis, may require a surgical referral.

Red flags should be directly asked to the patient in order to identify emergent situations [1, 2].

Physical Exam

Initial Setup to Optimize the Physical Exam

The physician should have the patient adjust the camera so the area of concern can be appropriately visualized. There should be enough space and appropriate positioning for adequate examination. The physician and patient should have appropriate lighting to see the other. The patient should wear proper clothing revealing the area of interest. The idea outfit would be a tank top, shorts, and sports bra for females. The patient and physician should be in a private area.

Inspection

The physician should ask the patient or someone to assist the patient in raising the shirt and expose the thoracic spine. If possible, the physician should view the spine in the coronal and sagittal views by having the patient rotate. In the sagittal view, the physician should note the degree of thoracic kyphosis and presence of pelvic tilt. The normal thoracic kyphosis ranges from 20° to 50°, with an average of 35°. In the coronal view, the physician should note symmetry between the shoulder levels, scapular positions, limb positions, level of the pelvis, thoracolumbar prominence, and any spinal curvature. In this view, the physician may also observe vertebral prominins, the most prominent upper back spinous process at C7. From here, the examiner can approximate how far down the back the pain is. In both views, changes in overlying skin and muscle bulk should be noted.

Palpation

Instruct patient to palpate with one finger over affected area then use deep palpation (if applicable).

Active Range of Motion

Range of motion of the neck and back should be assessed while the patient is standing. The patient will move to their end range of motion in flexion, extension, side-bending, and rotation of the neck and lower back. In an adolescent, assess for thoracic prominence (rib hump).

Neurological Examination

The physician should begin by assessing gait. There should be enough room for the patient to walk both towards and away from the camera with a full-body view. A second person may need to control camera placement.

Muscle strength testing should be performed for the neck and back. To assess muscle strength, a variety of maneuvers can be performed. Triceps chair push up can be used to assess strength of the triceps. A double leg squat and rise is a good general screen of quadriceps and lower extremity strength. Specific muscles can be targeted by having the patient move against gravity and with the addition of common household items of known weights. For example, a patient may use a gallon of milk, dumbbell, or heavy book for bicep curls or wrist flexion and extension. A tennis ball can be squeezed repetitively to assess grip strength. Deficits at T1 may lead to hand weakness.

Reflex testing may be challenging but can be attempted using the edge of a smartphone, side of the hand, or rubber-headed spatula. The physician should demonstrate and explain the maneuver for the patient to repeat.

Sensation testing is difficult. The patient can demonstrate where he or she feels numbness or paresthesia. Additionally, household items, such as a cotton ball and q tip can be used to assess small and large fiber modalities.

Consider examination of the shoulder if complaint originates in the upper thoracic spine and the hip if in the lower thoracic spine [2, 3].

Differential Diagnosis

The differential diagnosis for thoracic back is broad due to close proximity of visceral organs, the rib cage, and the many layers of muscle in the thoracic spine. Etiologies range from benign musculoskeletal injury to malignancy or life-threatening infection.

The majority of acute back pain complaints will resolve without intervention, but recurrence is common. Findings on initial assessment of back pain does not determine the long-term disability for the patient. Another contributing factor to the difficulty in managing back pain is anatomic findings on imaging may not correlate with the clinical picture and are not predictors of long-term pain. Therefore, the physician should rely on clinical findings over structural findings on imaging [4].

The differential diagnosis should be divided based on two methods. The first method of organization depends on type of pain: axial, referred, radicular, or chronic pain. The differential diagnoses may also be organized based on mechanical, nonmechanical, and visceral causes.

Axial back pain is localized to the same region as the affected part of the spine and becomes more intense with movement of the part or direct palpation. The patient will describe axial pain as achy, consistent, with quality ranging from sharp to dull. This type of pain occurs due to excitation of the nociceptive sensory neurons innervating the spine musculoskeletal structures surrounding the spine. Specifically, these nociceptor nerve endings can be found in the muscles and ligaments surrounding the spine, the periosteum of the vertebral body, the capsule of the apophyseal joints, and the annulus fibrosis of the intervertebral disc.

Referred pain differs from axial pain in quality and location. Patients will describe referred pain as a deep, dull pain that is projected between two sites. One location is the site of injury, and the other is an embryologically related site. For example, lumbar spine pain can refer to the musculature of the hip. This pain is described as referred pain, unless it follows the pathway of a spinal nerve, in which case it would be described as radicular pain. A separate type of referred pain is from a visceral organ to a somatic site, described in the visceral pain section below.

Radicular pain originates in the spine and follows the distribution of a spinal nerve, or along a dermatome. Patients with radicular pain vary in description of the pain and may have motor symptoms, including weakness, atrophy, and fasciculations.

Chronic pain often occurs in the absence of a clear precipitating factor. Pathologies such as degenerative disc disease or disc herniation may lead to a repetitive microtrauma and over time results in repetitive firing of nociceptive fibers, altered local pH, and a release of inflammatory molecules, such as cytokines, leukotrienes. This leads to central sensitization, from the repetitive depolarization of the sensory neurons and lowering of the excitatory threshold causing pain perceived with normal activities of daily life.

Mechanical Causes of Thoracic Spine Pathology

Vertebral compression fractures may be traumatic or nontraumatic. Patients who suffer traumatic vertebral compression fractures will likely present to the emergency department after their trauma and will not be seen in the telemedicine setting. Atraumatic vertebral compression fractures occur in patients on prolonged steroids or suffering from osteopenia or osteoporosis and occur from a fall of standing height or less, without major trauma such as a motor vehicle accident. These fractures most commonly occur in the midthoracic region (T7–T8) spine and the thoracolumbar junction (T12–L1). If a patient suffers from an osteoporotic vertebral compression fracture due to an acute event, he or she will more likely complain of acute back pain. Even sudden bending, coughing, lifting, or going over a speed bump can precipitate an acute fracture. Without an acute event, osteoporotic vertebral compression fractures may occur slowly over time and present as asymptomatic. If the patient is symptomatic, the pain will likely be localized to the midline spine and refer to the unilateral or bilateral flanks. If a nerve root or the spinal cord becomes compressed by the retropulsed bone fragments, the patient may experience radicular pain. Patients commonly experience height loss and kyphosis due to vertebral compression fractures [5].

Adult spinal deformity is becoming more common as the population of the world is staying active and living longer. This condition is defined as the group of conditions in which the spine bends abnormally to the right or left. Development of a spinal curve in childhood or adolescence is known as scoliosis. Patients who present for an adult spinal deformity can be divided into five categories. The first category is patients who have progression of their childhood or adolescent scoliosis. The four main causes of adult spinal deformity without history of childhood scoliosis include osteoporosis leading to collapse of the vertebrae, osteoarthritis, a specific focal problem such as degenerative disc disease or spondylolisthesis, and history of a spinal surgery that accelerated degeneration of the spinal column. These deformities can be asymptomatic but may also present with pain and disability.

Hyperkyphosis is a type of adult spinal deformity defined as excessive curvature of the thoracic spine. Thoracic kyphosis is measured by Cobb angle. As age increases, the thoracic kyphosis tends to increase due to multiple factors, including degenerative changes, vertebral compression fractures, muscular weakness, and altered biomechanics. Vertebral compression fractures are believed to be an important factor because there is a greater degree of thoracic kyphosis seen in patients with a history of vertebral fracture. Degenerative disc disease also is a major contributor in older adults because as disc desiccates in the aging process, the disc experiences asymmetrical height loss. More height is lost in the anterior segment, resulting in wedging and increased kyphosis. Pelvic tilt, lumbar lordosis, and cervical lordosis are both affected by the Cobb angle, leading to further disability and global spinal malalignment. There is an increased risk of falls due to the wider stance, slower gait velocity, and worse balance that result from hyperkyphosis. Pulmonary function is affected in patients with a higher degree of Cobb angle. An increase in the Cobb angle is associated with a decreased force vital capacity.

The most common type of idiopathic hyperkyphosis is Scheuermann's disease, which is described as a developmental disease of early adolescence resulting in anterior wedging of the vertebrae and subsequent hyperkyphosis. Genetic conditions associated with early onset hyperkyphosis include Marfan Syndrome, Ehlers–Danlos syndrome, osteogenesis imperfecta, and mucopolysaccharides [6–8].

Disc herniations most commonly occur at L5–S1 but can occur at any disc in the spine. The thoracic spine is the least common site. Herniation is classically defined as tearing of the annulus fibrosis of a disc, allowing extrusion of the nucleus pulposus secondary to trauma or degeneration. In patients with disc degeneration, even a benign stress such as a cough can result in herniation. This is because as the disc generates over time, the annulus fibrosis is weakened and a smaller force results in expulsion of the nucleus pulposus. Axial pain results from stimulation of the sensory innervation in the annulus fibers. Radicular pain may occur if the nucleus pulposus impinges on the surrounding neurologic structures. If the spinal cord is impinged, patients may present with myelopathy. Therefore, a careful motor and neurologic exam should be performed. Imagining is helpful in symptomatic patients, but the physician must be cautious because degenerative changes are often found on imaging in asymptomatic individuals. Most commonly, degenerative changes occur in the thoracolumbar junction which is anatomically located at T12–L1. A recent study has shown that segmental loads and more severe disc degeneration occurs superior to the anatomic thoracolumbar junction in patients without congenital disease or prior surgery occurs at T9–11 than T11–L1 [9].

Spondylosis refers to widespread degenerative or osteoarthritic changes in the spinal canal causing spinal stenosis. Stenosis is narrowing of a bony opening through which something travels. Spinal stenosis is narrowing of the central canal. Foraminal stenosis is narrowing of the intervertebral foramen. Both can lead to pain. Narrowing of the intervertebral foramen and central canal may result from a number of etiologies, including osteophytes, thickening of the ligamentum flavum, disc herniation, and spondylosis. In the thoracic spine, spinal stenosis can cause spinal cord compression and myelopathy, and foraminal stenosis can cause radiculopathy.

There are many muscles that course through the thoracic spine that are postural muscles and trunk stabilizing muscles. Each of these can develop myofascial pain secondary to postural abnormalities and overuse. The most common muscles that would cause pain in the thoracic spine region are periscapular from kyphotic and protracted shoulders. Symptoms of myofascial pain include tenderness in the muscle belly, erythema, trigger points, and muscular spasms. Myofascial pain may not be limited to one muscle, but often affects a group of muscles. Interspinous ligamentous strain may lead to focal pain in addition to myofascial pain [10].

The articulations between ribs and vertebral segments, known as costal facets, are unique to the thoracic spine. Costal facets are present on all vertebral bodies and transverse processes from T1–T9. The costal-vertebral articulation leads to increased rigidity in the spine. As a result, the thoracic spine is the most rigid part of the spine. The two main pathologies of the rib cage that may cause thoracic pain are costochondritis and costovertebral syndrome. Costochondritis is pain localized to the chest wall that is reproducible by palpation of the parasternal or costochondral joints. The costovertebral joint is a synovial joint within a synovial cavity, containing innervations, located where the head of the rib articulates with the vertebral body. Costovertebral pain will occur at this joint and mimic cardiopulmonary-related pain. Acceleration or deceleration injuries, blunt trauma, or overuse can lead to costovertebral pain. Costovertebral pain is a common complaint in ankylosing spondylitis. If a young male patient presents with a stooped posture due to costovertebral syndrome, ankylosing spondylitis should be considered on the differential [11–13].

Nonmechanical Causes of Thoracic Spine Pathology

There are four primary etiologies of nonmechanical thoracic spine pathology: malignancy, infection, rheumatic, or neurologic conditions. Red flag symptoms are aimed to promptly diagnose these conditions in order for the physiatrist to appropriately refer the patient.

Metastatic malignancy of the spine is more common than primary malignancy of the spine. The most common tumors that metastasize to the spine are from the breast, lung, and prostate. The most common primary tumors that affect the spine are lymphoma and multiple myeloma [14]. Rarely, malignancy of the spine is from a sarcoma. Pain from malignancy is constant and unimproved with rest. The patient may complain the pain is worse at night, or constant throughout. Unexplained weight loss, night sweats, increasing fatigue are all red flags that should raise a physician's concern for malignancy.

Infectious causes of pathology in the thoracic spine can be difficult to detect because the clinical presentation may be nonspecific. Patients may complain of nonspecific symptoms, including general malaise and fever, with back pain. Other patients may be asymptomatic except for pain in the thoracic spine. Physicians should have a high level of suspicion for infection in patients who have a history of documented sepsis, osteomyelitis, endocarditis, or other sources of infection that could spread to the vertebra or surrounding structures. Additionally, recent procedures such as injections, lumbar puncture, or spine surgery can introduce a pathogen to the vertebral column. Staphylococcal infections are most common. The pain in the thoracic spine will be subacute or chronic, exacerbated with movement, and the patient will have pain over the vertebrae when percussed on physical exam. If the infection is in close proximity to a nerve or nerve root, the patient may present with radicular symptoms. Infection may be identified as vertebral osteomyelitis, perivertebral abscess, or spinal epidural abscess on imaging. Even low suspicion of infection should be evaluated with urgent CT or MRI [15].

Rheumatologic conditions less commonly affect the thoracic spine but should be considered on the differential. Patients who present with involvement of multiple joint pain and inflammation in addition to spinal complaints should be considered for rheumatic disease. Rheumatoid arthritis rarely affects only the spine. However, seronegative arthropathies, such as ankylosing spondylitis, commonly present with back pain as the dominant symptom early in the disease. Ankylosing spondylitis is prominent in men, and often presents as lower back pain early in the diagnosis that progresses to stiffness. This may result in referred pain from the affected spinal level [16]. Psoriatic arthritis may also present with back pain.

Transverse myelitis is a type of myelopathy caused by inflammation of the spine. The patient will present with motor, sensory, and/or autonomic dysfunction that develops over hours to days. Sensory changes will usually present with dermatomal paresthesias with or without back pain at that associated level. Weakness typically affects the extensors of the arms and flexors of the legs. The most common autonomic symptoms are bladder and bowel dysfunction. The etiology of transverse myelitis is inflammatory, autoimmune, or infectious [17, 18].

Visceral Causes of Thoracic Spine Pathology

Visceral organs can cause referred back pain in the thoracic region. Pain sensing pathways in the spine converge nociceptive afferent somatic innervation and nociceptive afferent visceral innervation. Therefore, the patient is unable to differentiate these two types of pain in the central nervous system. In order to differentiate visceral types of back pain from musculoskeletal, the physician should take a detailed history. Visceral pathologies that may present as thoracic level back pain involve the stomach, specifically the posterior wall, such as peptic ulcer disease and malignancy in the stomach. Pathology involving the pancreas, such as pancreatic cancer, may also cause back pain. Depending on the anatomic location of involvement, the patient will have right-sided back pain if the head is involved and left-sided back pain if the tail or body are involved. Cholelithiasis may produce right-sided back pain as well. Kidney pathology, including malignancy, nephrolithiasis, and pyelonephritis, may also present with lower thoracic back pain that will radiate towards the groin. Retroperitoneal bleeding and. Abdominal aorta aneurysm may also present with pain at the thoracolumbar junction. Cardiac ischemia may commonly refer pain to the left of the thoracic spine and radiate to the shoulder. Atypically, cardiac ischemia will present with only mid thoracic back pain. Women are at higher risk for atypical presentations in general for cardiac ischemia [19, 20].

Special Considerations

Special considerations are important to ensure safety in advance, such as the need for an assistant or aid; especially for patients with cognitive deficits. If it is not possible to have an assistant or aid present, determine if the patient can safely perform a maneuver, if not defer the maneuver to when an in-person visit is feasible.

In patients who use wheelchairs or assistive ambulatory devices testing for gait and balance may have to be deferred for safety concerns unless there is an appropriate aid to provide guarded assistance. If the patient lives in a facility with on-site clinicians, consider communicating with the on-site provider during the telemedicine visit.

Limitations to the telemedicine visit when assessing the spine is the inability to assess for extremity reflexes such as the triceps, biceps, brachioradialis, patellar, Achilles reflexes or the pathologic reflexes such as the Hoffman's sign, Babinski reflex or clonus to assess for upper motor neuron damage. If the patient is not at a facility with on-site, clinicians manual muscle testing to evaluate for myelopathy would have to be deferred, unless the patient endorses sudden or progressively worsening weakness in the upper or lower extremities. In this case, send the patient to the emergency department for an in-person evaluation.

Tests that can be used to assess for myelopathy are the finger escape sign where the fingers are adducted and extended for 30 s. A positive result is ulnar drift and flexion of the fourth and fifth digits. The grasp and release test where the patient opens their palm, followed by gripping and releasing their fingers as many times as possible within a 10 s period. A positive result is the inability to complete 20 repetitions within 10 s. Another test is the 10-second step test where the patient is in a standing position and marches in place, raising the hips to 90 degrees of flexion. The provider records the number of alternating steps. A positive result is the inability to take 20 total steps within 10 s which could suggest an underlying myelopathy [21, 22].

Management/Treatment

Mechanical

Nineteen percent of patients who have a history of osteoporotic fracture will have another in the following year. Therefore, it is important to perform laboratory testing in order to identify the etiology. Secondary causes of osteoporotic vertebral fractures include hyperthyroidism, hyperparathyroidism, renal disease, Cushing's syndrome, and connective tissue disorders. If there are no neurologic deficits, suspected vertebral fracture can be evaluated radiographically with X-ray of the spine, which may demonstrate anterior wedging of one or more vertebrae with vertebral collapse, vertebral endplate irregularity, and if there is osteoporosis general demineralization. An underlying, destructive lesion from infection or malignancy, not osteoporosis, may result in posterior wedging of a vertebral fracture. The severity of fracture is staged radiographically based on height deformity.

Management of vertebral compression fracture begins with pain control and activity modification. Pharmacologic options for pain control are chosen based on severity of pain. Acetaminophen, naproxen, or ibuprofen are used for mild to moderate pain. If a trial of these analgesics does not improve the patients' pain and function, oral opioids may be used. Additionally, patients with moderate to severe pain may require opioids initially. If a patient has a history of gastrointestinal ulcers or bleeding, then NSAIDs are not the optimal pharmacologic treatment. Celecoxib, which is a specific NSAID which selectively inhibits COX-2, should not be used in patients with cardiovascular history. The most common opioid used for outpatient treatment of vertebral fracture is hydrocodone. Tramadol and other mixed analgesics may also be issued. Due to the side effect profile of opioids, a laxative should also be prescribed.

Complete bedrest is not recommended for patients with osteoporotic vertebral compression fracture because inactivity will result in further bone loss and deconditioning. Physical therapy should focus on gait and core strengthening, as tolerated. Hyperextension exercises may alleviate pain and prevent further kyphotic deformity. Important pearls for patient education include that pain should diminish gradually as activity tolerance increases and fractures may take 3 months to heal. Additionally, the most alleviating position for pain flares after activity is lying supine with hips and legs flexed. Bracing should only be used in the acute phases of treatment if it relieves the patient's pain. Risks of bracing include atrophy of core musculature with prolonged use may be required for patients who are incapacitated by pain due to vertebral fracture. Patients with vertebral compression due to osteoporosis should discuss further medical optimization, such as bisphosphonates, with their primary care provider. Neurologic abnormalities with vertebral compression fracture would require surgical evaluation and urgent CT or MRI should be performed. Vertebral augmentation procedures performed by a surgeon for vertebral compression fractures include vertebroplasty and kyphoplasty [5].

Posterior–anterior and lateral radiographs should be performed on patients with clinical signs of adult spinal deformity or scoliosis. From these, Cobb angles are measured to establish global, coronal, and sagittal alignment. Dynamic radiographs should also be ordered, including flexion extension, supine, and prone views. The dynamic views will assess the flexibility of the curve and the ability of the spine to compensate. Asymptomatic patients should be monitored for progression but do not require treatment. Deciding between non-operative or operative treatment for symptomatic patients is multifactorial, and therefore a physiatrist should be aware of the factors that make a patient appropriate for surgical referral. A trial of conservative management should be performed first, consisting of physical therapy, medications, and injections. Bracing is not recommended due to the risks of muscle deconditioning and atrophy. The T1 pelvic angle axis is a radiographic measurement useful in determining global alignment and sagittal balance. This measurement provides information from both the sagittal vertical axis and pelvic tilt, and therefore provides insight into the global spinal deformity and subsequent disability. The T1 pelvic angle overcomes the disadvantage posed by measures of sagittal deformity because the T1 pelvic angle is not diminished by compensatory mechanisms. Patients with loss of sagittal balance and an increased T1 pelvic angle are better candidates for surgical intervention, and therefore should be referred to a spine surgeon. Risk factors for poor surgical outcomes include tobacco use, pulmonary disease, coronary disease, vascular disease, diabetes, nutritional deficiency, increased body mass, osteoporosis, psychiatric disease, and lack of social support. Multiple studies have demonstrated that reconstructive surgery does improve quality of life. Therefore, once patients have failed conservative treatment, they should be referred to a surgeon for evaluation, who will make a decision based on the magnitude of symptoms and risks of intervention [8, 23].

Non-mechanical and Visceral Causes

Treatment by a physiatrist for these conditions should be coordinated with other physicians, such as a rheumatologist or primary care physician, to optimize multidisciplinary patient care.

CT or MRI can rule out a malignant or infectious process. If either is identified, prompt referral is required.

The initial evaluation of transverse myelitis should include clinical evaluation, physical exam, and a thorough history. The pattern of functional dysfunction may indicate a clear diagnosis. Common causes of transverse myelitis include multiple sclerosis, lupus, varicella-zoster virus, and tuberculosis. An MRI with contrast is the preferred imaging modality to rule out compressive myelopathy from abscess, hematoma, or herniated disc. Afterwards, a lumbar puncture will indicate if there are signs of inflammation and help determine the etiology [15].

Complications/Red Flags

Throughout the history and physical exam, the examiner should be assessing for red flags. If there are any red flag symptoms, the provider should escalate the patient's level of care. Any upper motor neuron changes or gait ataxia would indicate myelopathy. Progressive neurologic deficit is a red flag for expanding hematoma, abscess, or tumor causing a compressive myelopathy. Saddle anesthesia or bowel, bladder, and/or sexual dysfunction may indicate myelopathy or cauda equina syndrome. Fever and chills would indicate infection. Patients over 50 years old are at increased risk for malignancy and osteoporotic fractures. Malignancy often presents with night sweats and weight loss. Peptic ulcers can refer pain to the thoracic spine. Mechanical pain of the thoracic spine and visceral pain can mimic each other due to the shared afferent innervation of the autonomic nervous system, which originates from T1–L2 [24].

Follow-Up

After a telemedicine visit, an in person follow-up visit should be scheduled to assess examinations that were deferred during the telehealth visit. When new medications are prescribed close follow-up is necessary to assess its efficacy or the patient's response. Appropriate referrals for follow-up with other specialists should be provided when necessary.

References

1. Wang H, Ma L, Yang D, Wang T, Yang S, Wang Y, et al. Incidence and risk factors for the progression of proximal junctional kyphosis in degenerative lumbar scoliosis following long instrumented posterior spinal fusion. Medicine (Baltimore). 2016;95(32):e4443.
2. Woolf AD, Akesson K. Primer: history and examination in the assessment of musculoskeletal problems. Nat Clin Pract Rheumatol. 2008;4(1):26–33.
3. Laskowski ER, Johnson SE, Shelerud RA, Lee JA, Rabatin AE, Driscoll SW, et al. The telemedicine musculoskeletal examination. Mayo Clin Proc. 2020;95(8):1715–31.
4. Chou R, Huffman LH. Medications for acute and chronic low back pain: a review of the evidence for an American Pain Society/American College of Physicians clinical practice guideline. Ann Intern Med. 2007;147(7):505–14.
5. Rosen HN, Walega DR, Rosen CJ, Mulder JE. Osteoporotic thoracolumbar vertebral compression fractures: clinical manifestations and treatment. Waltham: UpToDate; 2019.
6. Diebo BG, Shah NV, Boachie-Adjei O, Zhu F, Rothenfluh DA, Paulino CB, et al. Adult spinal deformity. Lancet. 2019;394(10193):160–72.
7. Ailon T, Shaffrey CI, Lenke LG, Harrop JS, Smith JS. Progressive spinal kyphosis in the aging population. Neurosurgery. 2015;77(suppl_1):S164–72.
8. Good CR, Auerbach JD, O'Leary PT, Schuler TC. Adult spine deformity. Curr Rev Musculoskelet Med. 2011;4(4):159–67.
9. Murphy J, McLoughlin E, Davies AM, James SL, Botchu R. Is T9–11 the true thoracolumbar transition zone? J Clin Orthop Trauma. 2020;11(5):891–5.
10. Desai MJ, Saini V, Saini S. Myofascial pain syndrome: a treatment review. Pain Ther. 2013;2(1):21–36.
11. Erosa S, Erosa SC, Sperber K. Costovertebral pain syndromes. In: Musculoskeletal sports and spine disorders. Cham: Springer; 2017.
12. Waldman SD. Costovertebral joint syndrome. In: Atlas of common pain syndromes. Amsterdam: Elsevier; 2012.
13. McConaghy JR, Oza RS. Outpatient diagnosis of acute chest pain in adults. Am Fam Physician. 2013;87(3):177–82.
14. Heller J, Pedlow F Jr. Tumors of the spine: orthopaedic knowledge update. Spine. 1997;7:235–56.
15. Nussbaum ES, Rigamonti D, Standiford H, et al. Spinal epidural abscess: a report of 40 cases and review. Surg Neurol. 1992;38(3):225–31.
16. Brent LH. Inflammatory arthritis. Postgrad Med. 2009;355(19):2012–20.
17. West TW. Transverse myelitis—a review of the presentation, diagnosis, and initial management. Discov Med. 2013;16(88):167–77.

18. West TW, Hess C, Cree BAC. Acute transverse myelitis: demyelinating, inflammatory, and infectious myelopathies. Semin Neurol. 2012;32(2):097–113.
19. McLeod J. The physiology of visceral sensation and referred pain. Aust N Z J Surg. 1961;30(4):298–305.
20. Klineberg E, Mazanec D, Orr D, et al. Masquerade: medical causes of back pain. Cleve Clin J Med. 2007;74(12):905–13.
21. Satin AM, Lieberman IH. The virtual spine examination: telemedicine in the era of COVID-19 and beyond. Glob Spine J. 2020;11(6):966–74. https://doi.org/10.1177/2192568220947744.
22. Iyer S, Shafi K, Lovecchio F, et al. The spine physical examination using telemedicine: strategies and best practices. Glob Spine J. 2020;12(1):8–14. https://doi.org/10.1177/2192568220944129.
23. Protopsaltis T, Schwab F, Bronsard N, Smith JS, Klineberg E, Mundis G, et al. The T1 pelvic angle, a novel radiographic measure of global sagittal deformity, accounts for both spinal inclination and pelvic tilt and correlates with health-related quality of life. J Bone Jt Surg Am. 2014;96(19):1631–40.
24. Engstrom JW. Back and neck pain. In: Kasper DL, editor. Harrison's principles of medicine. 16th ed. New York: McGraw-Hill; 2005. p. 94.

The Telemedicine Lumbar Spine Exam

Rebecca Freedman, Jonathan Lee, and David A. Spinner

Low back pain (LBP) is one of the most common musculoskeletal complaints seen by healthcare professionals. Patients who present with LBP require a thorough, detailed assessment to help guide the practitioner through a multitude of differential diagnoses. The framework we outline assists in the standardization of a virtual lumbar spine exam. By following this format, providers can optimize the quality and efficiency of the virtual visit. We recommend providing the patient with instructions prior to the visit, including videos, diagrams, and a list of required items.

History

Obtaining the patient's history is arguably the largest component in understanding and managing LBP. When conducting any history with regard to LBP, it is imperative to ask questions pertaining to "red flag" symptoms. For instance, the provider should collect information about personal or family cancer histories, rheumatologic disorders, saddle anesthesia, or bowel or bladder

R. Freedman (✉) · J. Lee · D. A. Spinner
Department of Rehabilitation and Human Performance, Mount Sinai Hospital, New York, NY, USA
e-mail: Rebecca.Freedman@mountsinai.org;
Jonathan.Lee4@mountsinai.org; david.spinner@mountsinai.org

© The Author(s), under exclusive license to Springer Nature Switzerland AG 2023
M. Zakhary et al. (eds.), *Telemedicine for the Musculoskeletal Physical Exam*, https://doi.org/10.1007/978-3-031-16873-4_6

incontinence. Further questioning about fevers, night sweats, weight loss, pain that is worse at night or when lying supine, history of recent bacterial infection, IV drug use, and recent travel may be relevant. History collection should also involve the onset of symptoms and any traumatic events or mechanism of injury. The provider should ask further questions detailing the location and quality of the pain, if the pain radiates, what exacerbates the pain, and what relieves it. Acquiring an understanding of what the patient has tried in the past can provide clues towards navigating the telemedicine exam. This information can be gathered prior to the visit.

Physical Exam

The telemedicine lumbar spine exam is best performed with a specific setup and adequate space. We recommend providing the patient with examples and instructions for camera setup when the appointment is scheduled to minimize technical difficulties.

First and foremost, as with other telemedicine exams, make certain to explain to the patient that they should be in a comfortable, quiet, and private setting. Explain to the patient that you too are sitting in a private area where no one else can view the exam.

We recommend the use of a laptop or tablet for the telemedicine appointment as they are easily portable. The device should be placed at an appropriate distance so the provider can visualize the patient from head-to-toe as they maneuver, about 10 feet away [1]. The device may have to be adjusted during the visit to capture the patient at the best angle. Likewise, consider having enough room in your setup in order to demonstrate any movements or tests to help facilitate the visit.

Ensure the room has enough lighting, preferably natural light facing the patient. If natural light is not possible, lights placed behind the device are best. Try to have a blank wall behind the patient.

Ideally, the patient should wear shorts and a tank top or a sports bra. Hair should be pulled away from the shoulders, and the patient should be barefoot. We strongly encourage having another person participate in the encounter to assist the patient or adjust the camera as needed. The patient should have a chair, stool, yoga mat, cotton ball, safety pin, rubber spatula, or whatever props readily available.

Inspection

Inspection of the lumbar spine begins with observing the patient in both the coronal and sagittal planes. Patients should be observed from the front, side, and back views.

Anterior observation should assess head carriage, shoulder height symmetries, hip height differences, patellar alignment, and lower limb positioning (i.e., valgus or varus misalignment, or ankle pronation or supination) [2].

Next, have the patient turn their side towards the camera, revealing their lower back. Assessing the patient in the sagittal plane, check the patient's posture. Observe for an increase or decrease in both thoracic kyphosis and lumbar lordosis. Visually apply a plumb line, recalling that it normally falls from the external auditory meatus through the acromion and travels behind the hip and in front of the knee and ankle [3].

Have the patient turn their back towards the camera. An assistant may help expose the lumbar spine region. Posterior observation entails inspection of the spine, surrounding bone structures, and soft tissues. Note any gross abnormalities or deformities. Take note of any skin markings or lesions. If needed, the patient can move closer to the camera for visualization of any irregularity. Look for any muscle wasting or changes in muscle bulk. Take note of any atrophy or fasciculations throughout the spine and lower extremities [3].

Using bony landmarks, assess structural alignment and symmetry. Observe the iliac crests and posterior superior iliac spines (PSIS) for innominate symmetry. Instruct the patient to rest both of their hands on their "hip" bones (superior iliac crests) with their thumbs pointing towards their spine. This marks the L4–L5 interspinous level. After observing iliac crest height, guide the patient or their assistant towards the PSIS, using one finger on either side to locate. Comparing the heights of the iliac crests and PSIS may identify pelvic obliquity, which could indicate a leg length discrepancy or perhaps scoliosis [2]. The patient can be instructed to flex their trunk forward to reveal a rib hump deformity.

Do not forget to take note of your patient's facial expressions, any rigid movements, or preferred positioning, as these provide valuable clues for your diagnosis and management [2].

Palpation

Ask the patient to point to where their maximum pain is located. Instruct the patient to show you where the pain travels to. Take note of the distribution of pain and/or paresthesias. Have the patient or assistant lightly palpate over the affected area followed by deep palpation. Guide the patient or assistant to other landmarks, such as the PSIS, ischial tuberosities, greater trochanters, spinous processes, or paraspinal musculature. Palpation of the paraspinal musculature can identify tender points or regions of muscle hypertonicity and spasm. Tenderness to palpation of the vertebrae should be carefully noted, and it may be suggestive of malignancy, compression fractures, or osteomyelitis [2].

Active Range of Motion

Active range of motion (ROM) should ideally be tested in the standing position. The patient will move through their end ROM in all planes, including flexion, extension, side bending, and rotation. Make sure you have ample space to demonstrate these movements for the patient. A web-based goniometer or computerized digital inclinometer can be used for measuring ROM.

Have the patient face sideways to assess flexion and extension. Instruct the patient to flex forward and reach their hands to the floor. The first 60 degrees of flexion come from the lumbar spine, with the remaining movement coming from the hip and hamstrings.

6 The Telemedicine Lumbar Spine Exam

This is important to gauge if limitation in range of motion is due to the lumbar spine or to hamstring tightness [2].

Then, instruct the patient to move their lumbar spine into extension end range. Take note which motion or range limitation is due to pain, or which movement elicits more pain.

To assess side bending, tell the patient to face the camera. Have the patient reach one hand to the ground, followed by the other. Note any pain or limitations in ROM. Next, instruct the patient to rotate one way followed by rotation the other way, again noting any pain or limitations in range of motion.

Gait

There should be ample, unobstructed space for a gait assessment. The patient will need room to walk towards the camera and away from the camera. An assistant is recommended to control the camera placement and capture a full body view. Assessing gait pattern can provide information about motor deficits and can dictate the safety of performing certain tests [4].

Assess the patient taking about 5–10 steps away from the camera, then turning clockwise, and walking back towards the camera. If needed, have the patient ambulate with their assistive device or if unsteady, have another person assist. Look for abnormalities in the stance or swing phase, such as Trendelenburg sign, valgus positioning, tilting, or a foot drop. You can also visualize a shuffling gait, a wide based or narrow gait, or an antalgic gait. If able, have the patient tandem walk to assess balance. The patient can perform this next to a wall for support.

Muscle Strength

Muscle strength testing can be performed in various ways based upon a patient's function, mobility, and balance. Reasonable judgment should be used when asking a patient to perform certain maneuvers. Examinations should be tailored to each individual's ability and function to determine if motor weakness exists. The provider should take note of perceived or reported difficulty, asymmetrical weakness, or imbalance [1].

Psoas

To assess hip flexor strength (L1–L3 nerve roots), have the patient stand. If needed, the patient can use a chair for balance. Ask the patient to lift one leg into a marching position, and hold. Repeat on the other side. Alternatively, the patient can sit in a chair, and attempt to lift one thigh into a marching position, followed by the other. The ability to raise the leg into a marching position indicates at least 3/5 in strength, and if performed with ease, most likely indicates at least 4/5 in strength [5].

Quadriceps

To assess quadricep strength (L2–L4 nerve roots), instruct the patient to perform a double-legged squat and rise, using a chair for support if necessary. Observe depth, symmetry, knee positioning, and balance. If the patient is able, you can instruct him or her to perform a single leg squat, or a single leg rise from a chair, to assess for subtle differences in quadriceps strength [3]. Alternatively, the patient can step up onto a stool with support. Presumably, if the patient can perform an adequate double legged or single leg squat, or step up onto a stool with control, strength is most likely a 5/5. If the patient can perform these tasks but not necessarily with ease, grade their strength a 4/5.

For patients who cannot perform these maneuvers, the patient can sit in a chair and perform a seated knee extension [4]. If the patient can perform a seated knee extension, grade the patient a 3/5.

Tibialis Anterior

The ankle dorsiflexors (L4 and L5 nerve roots) can be tested with heel walking. Ask the patient to stand on their heels. Patients can use the chair or wall for balance as necessary. If the patient can safely do this, have the patient walk on their heels. If the patient can stand on their heels with ease, grade the patient a 4/5. If able to walk in a dorsiflexed position, grade the patient a 5/5.

If the patient cannot perform either of these tasks, have the patient sit in a chair. Assess if the patient is able to maximally and actively dorsiflex their ankles and toes while seated. Grade the patient a 3/5 if able to complete this maneuver.

Extensor Hallucis Longus

To assess extensor hallucis longus strength (L5 nerve root), have the patient sit in a chair, and instruct him or her to pull their big toe towards their nose. An assistant can place a downward force on the patient's big toe. If the patient is able to extend against gravity, grade him or her a 3/5. If the patient can resist some force, grade the patient a 4/5. If the patient can resist force with ease, give the patient a 5/5.

Gastrocnemius-Soleus

To assess ankle plantarflexion strength (S1 nerve root), have the patient rise up onto their toes, using the chair or wall for balance as needed. If the patient can execute this task, grade their strength at least a 4/5. Assess if the patient can safely perform 10 toe raises on each side or perform toe walking. If the patient is able to do so with ease, grade their strength a 5/5.

If the patient cannot perform either of these tasks, instruct the patient to sit in a chair. Assess if the patient is able to maximally and actively lift their heel from the ground while seated. Execution of this task grades the patient a 3/5 in strength.

Gluteus Medius

For hip abductor strength testing, have the patient stand facing away from the camera. Instruct the patient to stand on one leg and look for any hip drop in the unloaded leg. Repeat on the other side. A positive Trendelenburg sign is indicative of weak gluteus medius muscles.

Reflex Testing

This portion of the exam can be challenging for patients and assistants to perform. Oftentimes, it is difficult to have patients fully relax, or anticipation may prompt an exaggerated response. We advise providers to interpret reflex findings with caution, as accurate testing can be difficult [3, 6].

Reflex testing can be performed using the edge of a smartphone, side of a hand, or a rubber-headed spatula [3, 6]. An assistant can also perform reflex testing. Demonstration of the maneuvers can be helpful.

For patellar reflexes, instruct the patient to sit in the chair with their knee extended past 90° and heel on the ground. Explain to the patient how to locate their patellar tendon. Have the patient attempt to elicit their reflex by striking below the patella with their chosen object.

For Achilles reflexes, the patient can sit with their legs crossed. Using one hand to dorsiflex the foot, instruct the patient to use their other hand to strike the Achilles tendon with their chosen object.

Sensation Testing

A cotton ball and safety pin can be used to test sensation. The patient can refer to an image depicting dermatomal distributions. If available, an assistant can perform this portion of the exam. It may also be helpful for the provider to demonstrate and point to certain locations for guidance. The sensory exam performed virtually can evaluate dermatomal versus diffuse sensory loss.

Before beginning, have the patient swipe the cotton swab on their cheek and explain to the patient that this is what you are referring to as a normal sensation. Ask the patient to then use the cotton swab to touch below their inguinal crease (L1), their mid-anterior thigh (L2), medial femoral condyle (L3), medial malleolus (L4), third metatarsal head (L5), and lateral heel (S1). Patients should perform each location on both legs, assessing for normal, altered or no sensation. The sensory exam can be repeated with pin-prick.

Special Testing

Seated Straight Leg Raise

Instruct the patient to remain seated and fully extend their knee on one side, placing their heel to the floor. Pain radiating down the leg with knee extension, or leaning back to avoid pain, indicates

L4–L5 or L5–S1 disc herniation. Repeat the exam on the other side. If positive, there is no need to perform this exam in the supine position.

Slump Test

Similarly set up to the straight leg raise, have the patient sit in a chair. Ask the patient to slump forward and flex the neck, tucking in their chin. Then, instruct the patient to extend one knee straight, looking for reproduction of radicular findings. Practice caution with this test in patients who exhibited lumbar pain with flexion during AROM testing.

Seated/Supine FABER

Instruct the patient to sit upright in a chair. Place one ankle on the opposing knee to flex, abduct, and externally rotate the leg. Instruct the patient to gently apply pressure downward on the knee towards the ground, while keeping their buttocks evenly placed on the chair. If this maneuver elicits pain posteriorly, it could suggest sacroiliac joint pathology. If this maneuver elicits pain in the groin, it could suggest intra-articular hip pathology. This same test can be performed if the patient is lying down supine.

Kemp's Test

Have the patient stand, using a wall or chair for support. Ask the patient to actively extend their back, and side bend and rotate to one side, to load the posterior elements. If radicular pain is reproduced, this could indicate nerve compression. If the pain reproduced is non-radicular, this could indicate facet pathology.

Standing Stork Test

Have the patient stand with their feet approximately one foot apart. The patient should hold a wall or chair for support if necessary. Instruct the patient to bend one leg at the hip and knee, lifting the foot off of the ground, and lean backwards slowly. A positive test will reproduce lower back pain on the patient's symptomatic side. Pain with this movement may suggest sacroiliac joint pathology or spondylolysis.

Prone Stork Test

In this modified exam, the patient will lay prone on a flat surface. Instruct the patient to rise up on their forearms to extend their lumbar spine. Pain at or near the lower lateral sacroiliac joint may suggest sacroiliac joint pathology. The patient can rise onto their hands to further extend the lumbar spine.

Reverse Straight Leg Raise

Instruct the patient to lay prone on a flat surface and bend one knee. Ideally, have an assistant gently grasp the patient's knee and ankle, lifting both up, as to extend the hip and stretch the femoral nerve. Reproduction of paresthesias down the anterior thigh is suggestive of upper lumbar radicular disease.

Alternatively, the patient can lay on their side. An assistant can bend the patient's top knee and draw his or her leg backwards to extend the hip, while stabilizing the pelvis with one hand. Be certain to distinguish radicular pain from a tight rectus femoris muscle.

Ely's Test

Instruct the patient to lay prone on a flat surface. Have the patient maximally bend one knee. An assistant could passively flex the knee for the patient. This exam is positive if the hip of the tested side rises from the table, suggesting a tight rectus femoris.

Supine Straight Leg Raise

Have the patient lay supine, facing sideways towards the camera. The patient will slowly raise a straight leg off the floor until pain is provoked. Estimate the angle at which the patient felt pain. A positive test is known to be between 30° and 70° when radicular pain is reproduced in the posterior leg, radiating below the knee. Be sure to ask the patient questions about their pain to differentiate radicular pain versus hamstring tightness. Of note, if the patient feels pain in their groin when actively raising their leg, this could be indicative of hip pathology. Repeat the exam on the other side. If lifting the asymptomatic leg causes radicular pain in the involved leg, this exam is considered positive (crossed straight leg raise test).

If an assistant is available, he or she can passively and gently raise the patient's straight leg to perform this test.

Supine FAIR

Ask the patient to lay supine on a flat surface. Instruct the patient to bend their hip and knee to about 60°, and cross their lifted leg over their straight leg, to drop their knee to the ground. Reproduction of radicular pain down the posterior thigh of the bent leg is suggestive of piriformis syndrome.

Modified Gaenslen's Test

The patient must be lying down on a flat, elevated surface, such as a bed or couch. Carefully instruct the patient to lay supine, so that one leg is hanging off the edge. This will extend the hip at the sacroiliac joint. Pain in the sacroiliac joint region on the side which the leg is hanging is a positive test.

Thomas Test

Have the patient lay supine on a flat surface. Instruct the patient to bend both of their knees to their chest and use their arms to draw their knees in. Ask the patient to extend one leg slowly to the ground while holding the other leg bent. If there is a lack of hip extension, so as the thigh is not parallel with the surface, or an increase in lumbar lordosis, this indicates a positive test for iliopsoas tightness.

Examination of Related Areas

When assessing lower back pain, it is always important to assess the rest of the spine along with the hips and lower extremities. Please refer to the respective chapters if the patient's history suggests associated pain or pathology in other related body parts.

Special Considerations

Telemedicine allows doctors to physically see things that otherwise would not be possible in a traditional visit. For instance, if a patient is complaining of back pain at work, you can ask the patient to show you how he or she sits at their desk, their ergonomic setup, and what kind of chair he or she is using. The provider can also assess what kind of bed the patient sleeps on, how the patient walks up and down stairs, how the patient lifts household objects, etc. If a patient is in severe, debilitating pain, telemedicine allows the patient to have a virtual visit in the comfort of their own home, without the burden of coming into the office and arranging transportation.

Follow-Up

After working through your differential diagnosis list, determine if the patient will need in-person follow-up, i.e., emergency treatment, imaging, or a procedure. Routine follow-up visits can continue virtually and can be scheduled as needed. Physical therapy exercises can also be taught to the patient virtually, with the benefit of the provider watching real-time and correcting maneuvers.

References

1. Iyer S, Shafi K, Lovecchio F, Turner R, Albert TJ, Kim HJ, et al. The spine physical examination using telemedicine: strategies and best practices. Glob Spine J. 2020;12(1):8–14. https://doi.org/10.1177/2192568220944129.
2. Woznica DN, Press JM. Physical examination of the lumbar spine and sacroiliac joint. In: Malanga GA, Mautner K, editors. Musculoskeletal physical examination: an evidence-based approach. 2nd ed. Amsterdam: Elsevier; 2016. p. 108–10.
3. Laskowski ER, Johnson SE, Shelerud RA, Lee JA, Rabatin AE, Driscoll SW, et al. The telemedicine musculoskeletal examination. Mayo Clin Proc. 2020;95(8):1715–31. https://doi.org/10.1016/j.mayocp.2020.05.026.
4. Yoon JW, Welch RL, Alamin T, Lavelle WF, Cheng I, Perez-Cruet M, et al. Remote virtual spinal evaluation in the era of COVID-19. Int J Spine Surg. 2020;14(3):433–40. https://doi.org/10.14444/7057.
5. Wessell NM. The virtual physical exam provider instructions. Department of Orthopedics at University of Colorado. 2020. https://www.ucdenver.edu/docs/librariesprovider65/telehealth/telehealth-spine-physical-exam%2D%2D-patient-instructions.pdf?sfvrsn=a0b514b9_2.
6. Boes CJ, Leep Hunderfund AN, Martinez-Thompson JM, et al. Primer on the in-home teleneurologic examination: a COVID-19 pandemic imperative. Neurol Clin Pract. 2021;11(2):e157–64. https://doi.org/10.1212/CPJ.0000000000000876.

The Telemedicine Shoulder Exam

Mariam Zakhary, Craig Silverberg, and Angela Samaan

The shoulder is structurally and functionally complex as it has vast mobility, greater than any other joint in the body. The shoulder girdle is composed of three bones—the clavicle, scapula, and proximal humerus. There are four articular surfaces that compose the shoulder—sternoclavicular, acromioclavicular, glenohumeral, and scapulothoracic. The glenohumeral joint, commonly referred to as the shoulder joint, is the principal articulation. Its capsule consists of a fibrous capsule, ligaments, and the glenoid labrum. Static joint stability is provided by the joint surfaces and the capsulolabral complex, with the dynamic stability by the rotator cuff muscles and the scapular rotators (trapezius, serratus anterior, rhomboids, and levator scapulae). Nonetheless, glenohumeral joint instability is frequently observed and the shoulder joint is the most commonly dislocated major joint in the body [1].

M. Zakhary · C. Silverberg (✉) · A. Samaan
Department of Rehabilitation and Human Performance,
Icahn School of Medicine at Mount Sinai, New York, NY, USA
e-mail: mariam.zakhary@mountsinai.org

© The Author(s), under exclusive license to Springer Nature Switzerland AG 2023
M. Zakhary et al. (eds.), *Telemedicine for the Musculoskeletal Physical Exam*, https://doi.org/10.1007/978-3-031-16873-4_7

The rotator cuff is composed of four muscles—the supraspinatus, infraspinatus, teres minor, and subscapularis. The supraspinatus muscle plays a role in stabilizing the head of the humerus, preventing it from slipping inferiorly. Furthermore, this muscle synergistically assists with shoulder abduction (primarily with initial abduction to 30°), along with the deltoid periscapular and trapezius muscles. Supraspinatus pathology is commonly diagnosed in patients presenting with shoulder pain, weakness, or instability. The subscapularis muscle facilitates internal rotation, and the infraspinatus and teres minor muscles assist in external rotation [1].

Scapular stability collectively involves the trapezius, serratus anterior, and rhomboid muscles. The levator scapulae and upper trapezius muscles support posture; the trapezius and the serratus anterior muscles help rotate the scapula upward, and the trapezius and the rhomboids aid scapular retraction [1].

In this chapter, we review the proper work-up to deciphering shoulder injuries during a telemedicine visit.

History

A standard pain history (onset, duration, palliation/provocation, quality, location, and radiation) is imperative in diagnosing shoulder pathology. In addition, questions about previous injuries, past surgeries, comorbidities, and pertinent family history aid in formulating an assessment and plan.

Physical Examination [2, 3]

Initial Setup

Have the patient adjust the camera and lighting so that the examiner can appropriately visualize the area of concern. Make sure there is adequate space for the patient to move the upper extremity in all directions. Proper clothing (i.e., tank top, halter top, or sports bra) should be worn by the patient in order to ensure adequate visualization of the shoulder joint and its surrounding anatomy. Lastly, make sure privacy is maintained throughout the encounter, for both the patient and the examiner.

Inspection

Before focusing on the shoulder, note the patient's posture in both a seated and standing position. Once the patient has exposed the upper trunk and extremities, carefully inspect the front, the back, and the side of both shoulders. Important aspects include structural alignment (i.e., shoulder heights), changes in overlying skin, scars, effusion, erythema, ecchymosis, muscle atrophy, and scapular positioning.

Palpation

Have the patient point to the most painful spot with one finger. Then, have the patient palpate the following structures: the sternal notch, SC joint, clavicle, AC joint, long head of the biceps tendon, subacromial bursae, greater and lesser tuberosities of the humerus, coracoid process, and supraclavicular fossa. The examiner should monitor patient response as these areas are palpated first gently then more deeply as tolerated.

Range of Motion (ROM)

Test the active range of motion of both shoulders in cardinal views while the patient is either in a standing or sitting position. A web-based goniometer may be used.

Apley Scratch Test
Have the patient reach behind the back in internal rotation and behind the neck in adduction and external rotation. The degree of rotation can be quantified by documenting the level of the spinous process that can be reached.

Flexion
Starting with the patient having the forearm fully extended at the elbow with the arm attached to the side of the trunk, ask the patient to flex the arm at the shoulder by moving the upper extremity anteriorly and then superiorly, until it is above the head.

Extension
Starting with the patient having the forearm fully extended at the elbow and the palms supinated, ask the patient to extend both arms at the shoulder by moving the upper extremities posteriorly.

Abduction
Have the patient abduct both arms by bringing them laterally until they are above the head, at 180°.

Adduction
Have the patient flex the upper extremity forward to 90°. From this position, ask the patient to maximally adduct the shoulder by moving the arm horizontally all the way to the other side. Make sure to test one side at a time.

External Rotation
Have the patient flex the elbow at 90° with the arm attached to the trunk and the palms supinated. Then have the patient externally rotate the shoulder by bringing the forearms laterally.

Internal Rotation
Have the patient flex the elbows at approximately 45° with the fists clenched and the thumbs up. Then have the patient bring both hands behind the back until the thumbs touch the inferior aspect of the scapula.

Special Considerations for ROM
For a young child, you may need to ask them to reach for a toy in each plane or ask the parent to assist with passive range of motion.

Muscle Strength

Test muscle strength against gravity and with the addition of common household items of known weights or an additional person, if possible. After each resistance maneuver, ask the patient if the maneuver is painful or if the patient feels weaker than normal with these movements.

Special Tests [3]

Supraspinatus

Empty Can Test
Have the patient abduct the arm to 90° with neutral rotation. Then have the patient internally rotate the shoulder and angle forward 30°: the thumb should be pointing toward the floor. Have the patient self-resist a downwardly directed force to the arm. This test is positive if the patient experiences pain or weakness with resistance.

Drop-Arm Test
Have the patient abduct their shoulder to 90°. Then have the patient slowly lower the arm to the side in the same arc of movement. This test is positive if the patient is unable to return the arm to the side slowly or has severe pain when attempting to do so.

Serratus Anterior

Standing Push-Up Test
Have the patient flex both arms to 90° against the wall. This test is positive if there is winging of the scapula at the medial border.

Shoulder Impingement

Hawkins Test
Have the patient flex the shoulder to 90°, flex the elbow to 90° and internally rotate the forearm. This test is positive if pain is elicited below the AC joint.

Acromioclavicular Joint

Scarf Test
Have the patient flex the shoulder to 90°, flex the elbow to 90° and then cross adduct the shoulder, resting the hand on top of the contralateral shoulder. This test is positive if pain is elicited over the AC joint.

Biceps Tendinopathy

Speed's Test
Have the patient fully extend the elbow, supinate the forearm, flex the shoulder to 60° and then apply self-resistance in a downward direction. The test is positive if pain is reproduced in the bicipital groove.

Yergason's Test
Have the patient flex the elbow to 90° and pronate the forearm while keeping the arm at the side. Have the patient supinate the arm while applying self-resistance at the wrist. The test is positive if pain is reproduced in the bicipital groove.

Labral Tear (SLAP Lesions)

O'Brien's Test
Have the patient flex the shoulder to 90° with full elbow extension, combined with 10°–15° of shoulder adduction and maximal internal rotation. Have the patient apply self-resistance with a downward force to the tested arm. The test is repeated with supi-

nation. The test is positive for an SLAP lesion if pain provoked during the first testing position lessens or disappears during the second position.

Cervical Nerve Root Disorder

Spurling's Test
Have the patient extend and side bend the neck, and then apply axial compression with the opposite arm to the side causing problems. The test is positive if the pain or radiculopathy is reproduced.

Differential Diagnosis

Despite the multiple musculoskeletal diagnoses that can cause shoulder pain, it is important to rule out other diagnoses that may cause referred pain to the shoulder [4]. Other diagnoses to consider include proximal nerve impingement at the level of the cervical spine due to disc herniation or neural herniation and peripheral nerve entrapment distal to the spinal column with involvement of the long thoracic or suprascapular nerve [5]. Moreover, it is important to maintain a high index of suspicion in order to exclude life-threatening conditions. For example, a patient with myocardial ischemia may classically present with left shoulder pain. Other serious considerations include splenic laceration, ruptured ectopic pregnancy, superior pulmonary sulcus tumor, or gallbladder pathology [4, 5]. A careful history and examination will help decipher intrinsic shoulder pain from referred shoulder pain.

Management/Treatment

When history and examination support a musculoskeletal cause for shoulder pain, radiologic evaluation may be warranted to further assess the cause of symptoms. A variety of imaging studies are appropriate in different circumstances. Plain film radiography is usually the first imaging modality for most shoulder pathology [6]. Ultrasonography is a safe, noninvasive tool that may be useful in evaluating shoulder anatomy including the rotator cuff muscles, biceps tendon, subacromial–subdeltoid bursa, and calcific deposits [7]. Computer tomography (CT) is useful for evaluation of fracture or displacement pathology. Use of intravenous contrast is reserved for evaluation of soft tissue and for suspected bone tumor or abscess [8]. When evaluating soft tissues of the shoulder, magnetic resonance imaging (MRI) is the main modality. Similar to CT, MRI with intravenous contrast is reserved for evaluation of soft tissue and for suspected bone tumor or abscess [9]. Radionuclide bone scan is generally limited to evaluation of infection or suspected metastases [6]. Arthrography uses fluoroscopic guidance to facilitate installation of contrast into the joint in order to identify pathology within the joint [10].

Pain control to achieve early return to normal function is the cornerstone of treatment. Patients should be instructed to avoid aggravating activities [11]. NSAIDs and non-opioid analgesics may often alone help achieve adequate pain relief. It is important to advise patients on side effects and contraindications to NSAID use including gastrointestinal bleeding and renal impairment [11, 12]. There is evidence that suggests short-term benefit of physical therapy for shoulder pain. There is no evidence on the best time for referral to physical therapy; however, early referral can be advisable in more severe cases [13]. Modalities such as electrical stimulation, phonophoresis, iontophoresis, and therapeutic ultrasound may be used to aid in pain relief. Oftentimes, directions for home exercises can be sufficient [11]. If symptoms persist despite these options, glucocorticoid injections may be reasonable. Surgery may be indicated in patients who fail both pharmacologic and nonpharmacologic therapy [5].

Complications/Red Flags

Urgent investigations and/or referral to secondary care may be warranted in patients who present with acute symptoms (particularly pain that restricts all passive and active range of motion) with a history of trauma, systemic symptoms (such as fever, night sweats, weight loss), abnormal joint shape, local mass or swelling, local erythema over a "hot" and tender joint, and severe restriction of shoulder movement [5, 12]. It is important to further evaluate a patient's history, particularly asking about other systemic conditions that may lead you to an alternate diagnosis.

Follow-Up

There is no clear evidence on the best time to follow-up with patients presenting with shoulder pain. It is reasonable to advise patients with shoulder pain to follow-up within 2 weeks of initiating therapy with further recommendation to follow-up sooner if symptoms acutely worsen [12].

References

1. Malanga G. Musculoskeletal physical examination. Amsterdam: Elsevier; 2016.
2. Laskowski ER, et al. The telemedicine musculoskeletal examination. Mayo Clin Proc. 2020;95(8):1715–31.
3. "Musculoskeletal/Orthopaedics." *Physiopedia*. www.physio-pedia.com/Category:Musculoskeletal/Orthopaedics.
4. Johnson TR. The shoulder. In: Snider RK, editor. Essentials of musculoskeletal care. Rosemont: American Academy of Orthopaedic Surgeons; 1997.
5. Mehta S, Gimbel JA, Soslowsky LJ. Etiologic and pathogenetic factors for rotator cuff tendinopathy. Clin Sports Med. 2003;22:791.
6. Willick SE, Sanders RK. Radiologic evaluation of the shoulder girdle. Phys Med Rehabil Clin N Am. 2004;15:373.
7. Lew HL, Chen CP, Wang TG, Chew KT. Introduction to musculoskeletal diagnostic ultrasound: examination of the upper limb. Am J Phys Med Rehabil. 2007;86:310.
8. Haapamaki VV, Kiuru MJ, Koskinen SK. Multidetector CT in shoulder fractures. Emerg Radiol. 2004;11:89.
9. Opsha O, Malik A, Baltazar R, et al. MRI of the rotator cuff and internal derangement. Eur J Radiol. 2008;68:36.
10. Rhee RB, Chan KK, Lieu JG, et al. MR and CT arthrography of the shoulder. Semin Musculoskelet Radiol. 2012;16:3.

11. Dela Rosa TL, Wang AW, Zheng MH. Tendinosis of the rotator cuff: a review. J Musculoskelet Res. 2001;5:143.
12. Rees JD, Wilson AM, Wolman RL. Current concepts in the management of tendon disorders. Rheumatology (Oxford). 2006;45:508.
13. Page MJ, Green S, McBain B, et al. Manual therapy and exercise for rotator cuff disease. Cochrane Database Syst Rev. 2016;2016:CD012224.

The Telemedicine Elbow Exam

Mariam Zakhary, German Valdez, and Monica Gibilisco

In this chapter, we will discuss the physical examination of the elbow via tele medicine. Beginning with patient history, going through the physical exam itself, and concluding with differential diagnosis and management.

Chief Complaint/Patient History

The clinician should take a detailed history of the elbow pain. This should include duration, intensity, severity, presence of radiation, presence of neurological symptoms, aggravating and alleviating factors, and previously attempted therapies. In addition, one should note the patient's occupation, history of trauma, surgical history, and general medical history.

M. Zakhary
Department of Rehabilitation Medicine, Mount Sinai Hospital,
New York, NY, USA
e-mail: mariam.zakhary@mountsinai.org

G. Valdez (✉) · M. Gibilisco
Department of Rehabilitation and Human Performance, Mount Sinai,
New York, NY, USA
e-mail: german.valdez@mountsinai.org;
monica.gibilisco@mountsinai.org

© The Author(s), under exclusive license to Springer Nature
Switzerland AG 2023
M. Zakhary et al. (eds.), *Telemedicine for the Musculoskeletal Physical Exam*, https://doi.org/10.1007/978-3-031-16873-4_8

Physical Exam

Initial Setup

Place the camera at approximately 4–5 feet off the ground, which for many is about the height of a table or counter. Have the patient stand approximately 6 feet away from the camera. Have the patient adjust the camera so the physician can appropriately visualize the elbow, the proximal arm, and the distal forearm [1].

As with every examination, ensure proper lighting for the room, along with sufficient space.

Ask the patient to wear a short sleeve shirt, tanktop, or any other top without sleeves. Long sleeves which roll past the elbow make adequate examination difficult.

Inspection/Observation

Visually inspect the elbow joint structural alignment, and for any signs of asymmetry, take note of the muscle contour.

Observe for any skin changes such as effusion, erythema, or ecchymosis. Also look for scars, occupational injuries, signs of physical abuse and drug use. Take particular note of the muscle mass of the surrounding muscles, such as the triceps, biceps, and forearm muscles. An example of biceps tendon tear (Fig. 8.1).

Palpation

Ask the patient to point, with one finger, the area of maximal pain. And then proceed to palpate over the affected area. Afterwards ask the patient to palpate the medial, lateral, and posterior bony aspects of their elbow; reporting pain when felt.

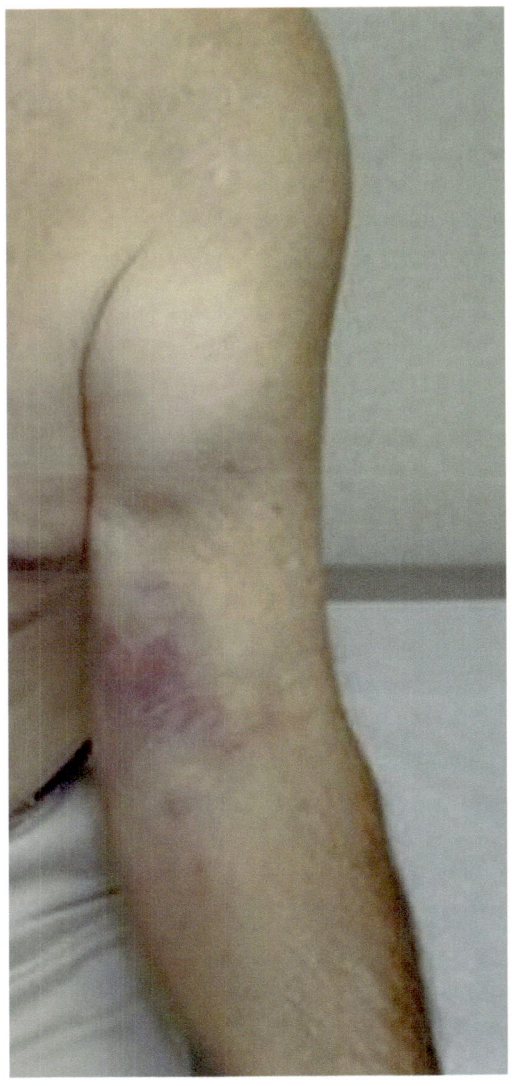

Fig. 8.1 Biceps tendon tear [2]

Active Range of Motion

For flexion and extension, ask the patient to face the camera and abduct the arms to 90°; with palms facing upward. Ask the patient to flex and extend their arm at the elbow. A web-based goniometer can be used to measure the range of motion (Fig. 8.2).

For supination and pronation, ask the patient to face the camera with arms adducted to their sides and elbows bent at 90°. A web-based goniometer can measure the range of motion by assessing hand/finger movement. Normal elbow range of motion values can be referenced at (Table 8.1).

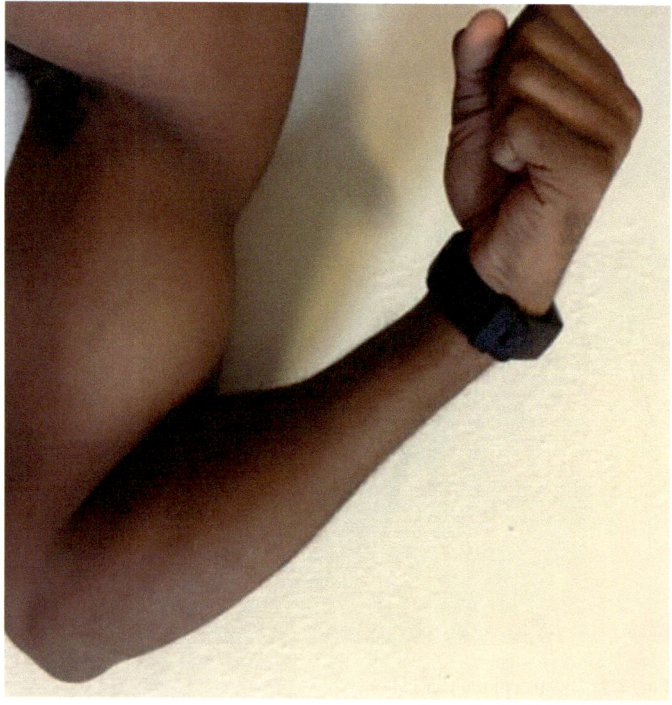

Fig. 8.2 Elbow flexion

Table 8.1 Normal range of motion of the elbow [3]

Movement	Degrees
Flexion	140–160
Extension	0–10
Pronation	80–90
Supination	90

Neurological Examination

Muscle Strength
Strength testing can be performed against gravity and with objects of known weights. Take note of the muscle contour of the bicep during flexion and the triceps during extension.

Reflex Testing
To elicit reflexes the clinician should demonstrate reflex testing for the patient by striking the opposite elbow. Both the triceps and biceps tendon reflex should be tested. Household objects can be used such as the side of the hand, a rubber headed spatula or using the edge of a smartphone [1].

Sensation
In order to test for sensation, ask the patient to follow the provider's lead and lightly press on five different points of the arm. Including the medial and lateral elbow, along with the palmar aspect of the first, third, and fifth digit. The patient should touch one point on one arm, and then compare the sensation on the contralateral arm.

Special Tests

The chair push-up test. Ask the patient to turn 90° with the injured elbow closest to the camera.

With the forearm in supination ask the patient to push off from a chair. This tests for posterolateral stability. Pain and/or apprehension during this maneuver would indicate a positive finding [4].

Provocative Lateral and Medial Epicondylitis Testing

Lateral epicondylitis: Ask the patient to repeatedly extend the wrist and supinate while holding a weighted object.

Medial epicondylitis: Ask the patient to repeatedly flex the wrist and pronate while holding a weighted object.

Examination of Related Areas

Please refer to Chaps. 8 (Shoulder Exam) and 10 (Hand and Wrist Exam), respectively, for additional details.

Considerations for Certain Populations

Acute Elbow Injuries in Children
Nursemaid's Elbow
- Usually caused by a sudden pull on a child's arm (typically ages 2–5 years old).
- Injury pathology is that the radial head is pulled out of the joint with the humerus, trapping one of the ligaments around the elbow.
- PE: Typically no swelling/erythema, but the child can only bend their arm slightly at the elbow and will be guarding.
- Reduction will have to take place in a hospital/doctor's office, but it is easily corrected with a simple maneuver.

Chronic Elbow Injuries in Children
Little League Elbow
- Overuse injury that is typically caused by repeating throwing in sports, without resting between throws.
- Overhead throwing causing the cartilage growth plate in children to become irritated.
- Pain can occur after one hard throw or gradually over the course of a baseball season.
- Swelling, redness of warm can be seen on the elbow.

- Treatment depends on extent of the injury to the growth plate but can range from rest and ice to cast or surgical pinning.
- Physical therapy is also crucial in these injuries once healing is complete to gradually return to throwing.

Osteochondritis Dissecans
- Occurs when lack of blood flow causes bone and cartilage to separate from the surface of a joint.
- Can occur suddenly due to trauma (e.g., fall) or over time from repetitive stress on a joint.
- Most common in athletic active children over age 10 (baseball pitchers, gymnasts, swimmers, quarterbacks).
- The repetitive motion with compressive forces across the lateral part of the elbow can cause a lot of pain and can lead to catching, locking, grinding, or a loss of motion.
- Treatment is typically resting, possible splint/cast and physical therapy.
- Slow progression back to the sport is essential with the help of a physical therapist to reduce the risk of future osteoarthritis to the joint [5].

Differential Diagnosis

The location and quality of elbow pain can generally localize the injury to one of the four anatomic regions: anterior, medial, lateral, or posterior.

Anterior Elbow Pain

Bicep's Tendinopathy
Inflammation of the tendon around the long head of the biceps muscle.

- History often includes repeated elbow flexion with forearm supination or pronation (dumbbell curls).

Physical exam = The Hook Test: Ask the patient to place the palm of his or her hand in front of their face as if you were reading a book. Try to hook the index finger of their opposite hand behind a cord (tendon) in front of your elbow. Pain can indicate biceps tendinopathy.

Medical Elbow Pain

Medial Epicondylitis (Golfer's Elbow)
Flexors and pronators of the wrist insert on the medial epicondyle. Repetitive flexion of the wrist (a golfer's swing) can cause pain and inflammation around this bony prominence.

Physical exam = pain after patient repeatedly flexes the wrist and pronates while holding a weighted object.

Ulnar Collateral Ligament Injury
Medial elbow tenderness and pain during the acceleration phase of motion.

- Occurs in athletes who play sports that involve overhead throwing (baseball, volleyball, javelin).
- Patients with an acute UCL injury usually report the sensation of a pop followed by the immediate onset of pain and bruising around the medial elbow.
- Key to diagnosis is assessment of the medial joint space laxity or instability against valgus forces. The medial joint space of the symptomatic elbow should be compared with the asymptomatic side for the amount of opening and the subjective quality of the end point while a valgus force is applied across the joint.

Physical Exam
Moving Valgus Stress Test: Patient should place the shoulder in 90° of abduction and external rotation. While constant valgus torque on the elbow is maintained, the elbow is quickly flexed and extended. A positive result is defined as pain between 70° and 120° degrees of flexion.

Cubital Tunnel Syndrome
Compressive or traction neuropathy of the ulnar nerve as it passes through the cubital tunnel of the medial elbow.

- The pain is usually associated with numbness and tingling in the ulnar border of the forearm and hand, and in the ring and little finger of the hand.
- Weakness of the intrinsic muscles of the hand may develop.
- Patients may have nighttime pain from sleeping with the elbow fully flexed.

Physical Exam
Tinel sign at the cubital tunnel: Ask patient to find the groove on the medial sign of the elbow, between the olecranon process and medial epicondyle, and repeatedly tap the groove using their other hands index finger. Reproduction of numbness/tingling is a positive sign.

Lateral Elbow Pain

Lateral Epicondylitis (Tennis Elbow)
Extensors and supinators of the wrist insert on the lateral epicondyle. Repetitive extension of the wrist (back hand motion in tennis) can cause pain and inflammation around this bony prominence. Lateral epicondylitis is actually 7–10× more common than medial epicondylitis.

Physical Exam = Pain after patient repeatedly extends the wrist and supinates while holding a weighted object.

Radial Tunnel Syndrome
Compressive neuropathy of the radial nerve.

- Pain in the lateral aspect of the elbow, and down the forearm and into the hand, without any motor symptoms.
- A history of repetitive forearm supination and pronation (twisting of the hand) (e.g., carpenters, mechanics).

Posterior Interosseous Nerve Syndrome

Compressive neuropathy of the posterior interosseous nerve, which is the deep branch stemming off the radial nerve.

Physical Exam = Middle Finger Test = Painless loss of the ability to extend the middle finger against resistance.

Posterior Elbow Pain

Olecranon Bursitis

Inflammation of the bursa over the olecranon.

- History could include trauma to the elbow or prolonged pressure on elbow (leaning on tabletop, plumbers who crawl on elbows and knees).
- Boggy nontender mass over the back of the elbow.
- If the bursa becomes infected, the skin becomes red, warm, painful.

Posterior Impingement

Impingement of the olecranon tip in the olecranon fossa, which may cause osteophyte formation and a fixed flexion deformity over time presents in younger athletes who perform repetitive valgus stresses while in hyperextension (i.e., javelin throwers).

Physical Exam

Posterior elbow pain when forced into full elbow extension.

Triceps Tendinopathy

Inflammation of the triceps tendon.

- Tenderness at the triceps insertion
- Pain at the posterior elbow with extensor use (pushing motions)
- Tenderness at the triceps insertion (AAFP)

Elbow Instability

Elbow locking, snapping, or subluxation when the elbow is extended and the forearm is supinated, i.e., a positive chair push-up test as above.

Management/Treatment

If history or physical exam is consistent with a history of trauma, arthritis, or loose fragments. Management typically begins with imaging such an X-ray.

As with many musculoskeletal injuries, once should follow a stepwise approach
1. Decreasing pain and inflammation
   (a) Tylenol
   (b) NSAIDS
   (c) Muscle relaxers
   (d) Modalities; heat and post activity icing
   (e) US guided local corticosteroid or platelet-rich plasma injection in refractory cases
2. Restoring normal symmetric range of pain
3. Normalize strength
4. Proprioceptive training
   +/− sport-specific training. Alter the mechanics leading to injury (depending on the patient)

Unique and Extra Considerations

Medial Epicondylitis
Stretching during the painful period is important. May use a tennis elbow counterforce strap.

Lateral Epicondylitis

Tennis elbow strap worn around the forearm, just distal to the elbow. Wrist splint to rest the common extensor tendons. A larger racquet grip and head and less string tension may be beneficial. PRP injection is more effective than steroid injection in refractory pain in medial epicondylitis [6].

Complications/Red Flags

Joint instability: Warrants surgical evaluation

Infection: Signs of infection include warmth, swelling, and erythema. Warrants fluid aspiration and culture.

Elbow dislocation: Often occurs posteriorly after a fall on an outstretched hand. Associated with fracture of the radial head, injury to brachial artery and median nerve, thus a thorough neurovascular evaluation is vital. Any deficit warrants immediate surgical evaluation. Complications include loss of ROM, ectopic bone formation, neurovascular injury, and elbow arthritis.

"Popeye Sign"—A deformity accompanied by swelling and ecchymosis. Suggestive of a biceps tendon avulsion. A tendon rupture and avulsion would require surgical intervention.

Follow-Up

After initial evaluation, it is important to provide follow-up within (4–6) weeks. Remember to provide sufficient referral to physical or occupational therapy as deemed warranted depending on the injury.

References

1. Laskowski ER, Johnson SE, Shelerud RA, et al. The telemedicine musculoskeletal examination. Mayo Clin Proc. 2020;95:1715–31.

2. https://orthoinfo.aaos.org/en/diseases%2D%2Dconditions/biceps-tendon-tear-at-the-elbow/.
3. Malanga GA, Nadler S. Musculoskeletal physical examination: an evidence-based approach. Maryland Heights: Elsevier Mosby; 2006.
4. Tanaka MJ, Oh LS, Martin SD, Berkson EM. Telemedicine in the era of COVID-19: the virtual orthopaedic examination. J Bone Jt Surg Am. 2020;102(12):e57. https://doi.org/10.2106/JBJS.20.00609.
5. Elbow Injuries. 2022. https://www.choa.org/medical-services/orthopaedics/injury-finder/elbow. Accessed 06 Dec 2020.
6. Shatzer M. Physical medicine and rehabilitation pocketpedia. 2nd ed. New York: Springer Publishing Company; 2012.

The Telemedicine Hand and Wrist Exam

9

Andres Arredondo, Hashem E. Zikry, and Amie M. Kim

The hand and wrist are highly functional, while the least protected and vulnerable to significant disability. A proper exam confers valuable information in the evaluation and management of high liability injuries. Anatomic knowledge is imperative for fully understanding the contribution of each structure with particular attention to the function of the muscles and tendons at each joint and the vascular and nerve supplies.

Chief Complaint/Patient History

The most common chief complaints for the hand and wrist include: pain, swelling, discoloration, deformity, stiffness, or loss

---

Photo Credit: John Conway, MD. Resident Physician, Icahn School of Medicine at Mount Sinai

---

A. Arredondo · H. E. Zikry (✉)
Department of Emergency Medicine, Icahn School of Medicine at Mount Sinai, New York, NY, USA
e-mail: Andres.ArredondoSantana@mountsinai.org;
hashem.Zikry@mountsinai.org

A. M. Kim
Department of Emergency Medicine, Physical Medicine Rehabilitation, Icahn School of Medicine at Mount Sinai at Beth Israel, New York, NY, USA
e-mail: amie.kim@mountsinai.org

© The Author(s), under exclusive license to Springer Nature Switzerland AG 2023
M. Zakhary et al. (eds.), *Telemedicine for the Musculoskeletal Physical Exam*, https://doi.org/10.1007/978-3-031-16873-4_9

of function. Additional questions include: occupation and athletic sport participation with recent change in activity load or type, inciting or provoking events, and history of predisposing medical conditions that may manifest in the upper extremities including neuropathy, vascular disease, inflammatory or auto-immune arthropathies, any prior injuries, or chronic disabilities.

Given the surface anatomy of the hand and wrist, identifying the location of pain is an important first step. The patient should demonstrate the site of maximal pain and any radiation. The provider can then ask the patient to establish if the pain is focal, or unilateral, identify the timeline when the pain first began and its progression, any preceding events, aggravating or relieving factors, severity on a scale of (1–10), daytime variation of pain, and additional pain patterns in reproducibility. Elucidate remedies the patient has tried including medication and time of last dose. As always, red flag symptoms must be eliminated. These include infection, neoplasm, vascular compromise. Questions include: night sweats, fever, pain out of proportion to exam, decreased range of motion, weight loss, numbness, weakness, duskiness, or discoloration at the fingertips.

Physical Exam

Initial Setup

Several aspects of the patient setup can be optimized to perform a detailed exam. First, the room should have adequate lighting, and be devoid of background clutter, distractions, or noise. Instruct the patient to remove clothing or accessories that cover the hands or wrists; including gloves, rings, and bracelets. An in-person hand exam is usually conducted with the patient seated facing the provider to visualize the patient's hands while also evaluating the response to exam maneuvers. Both hands should be visible in the field of view in order to compare and assess for symmetry. This is difficult to achieve in a video exam given the limited field of view and resolution obtained through most cameras. To prioritize visualization of the hands and wrist, the patient should sit and face the device's camera directly with a flat surface where the hands can

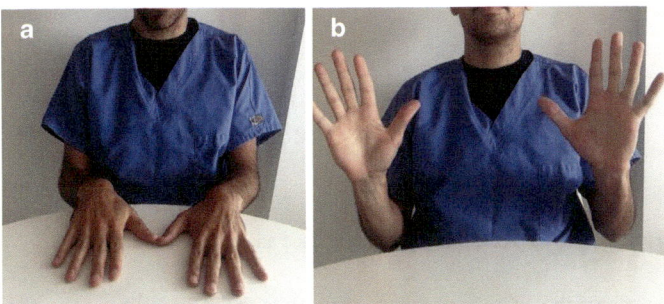

Fig. 9.1 (**a**, **b**) Patients faces the camera directly with a flat surface in resting (**a**) and raised (**b**) positions

rest (Fig. 9.1a). The camera's field of view can alternate between centered on the hands as they rest on the table, or on the patient's shoulders with the hands raised (Fig. 9.1b). This is best achieved with the use of an adjustable laptop camera. If a handheld device is utilized, a family member or friend can hold the device to visualize both patient's hands at all times.

Inspection/Observation

The first step of the exam entails inspecting the patient's hands and wrist as they move through a full range of pronation and supination. Both volar and dorsal aspects are evaluated. The most obvious pathology here includes gross deformities of the fingers such as a swan neck, mallet, or boutonniere contractures.

During inspection, include the entire forearm, elbow, upper arm, and shoulder. Identify changes in the overlying skin such as effusions, erythema, and ecchymosis. Visualize gross muscle atrophy, particularly in small hand muscles innervated by the median and ulnar nerves; the thenar, hypothenar, interossei, and lumbricals.

Palpation

Guide the patient in self-palpation of the anatomic structures of interest of the hand and wrist. The provider should use layman's

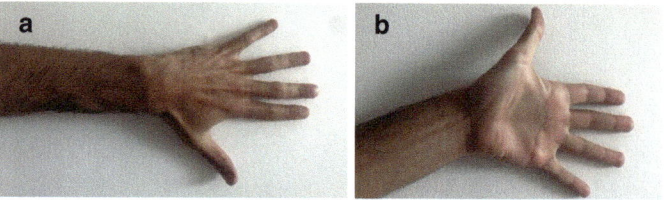

Fig. 9.2 (**a**, **b**) Descriptive terms of surface anatomy structures

terms of the surface anatomy (Fig. 9.2a, b). To facilitate, the provider can also demonstrate by palpating his own hands. The patient palpates the unaffected hand first and the affected side second to provide a comparison.

Palpation should be thorough, as the superficial structures of the hand and wrist can be very informative. The patient should note any difference in temperature between the two hands. A warm hand can indicate an infectious or inflammatory process, and ischemic pathology in a cooler hand. If available, a friend or family member can palpate the patient's hands for a more accurate comparison of temperature. Ask the patient to identify any "bumps" or "lumps" or areas of swelling and whether painful or painless. This assesses for nodules, masses, or fluctuance. Wrist effusions are typically identified at the dorsal aspect, and an occult effusion is further exaggerated with the wrist placed into passive dorsiflexion. The patient should note any areas of tenderness as they self-palpate and bring any area with positive findings into the camera's focus for the provider to better delineate relevant structures.

Motor Exam

Range of Motion

The first part of the motor examination of the hand and wrist consists of evaluating for range of motion (ROM) abnormalities. An approach has been previously described by [1]. The patient uses the contralateral hand to demonstrate passive ROM of the affected

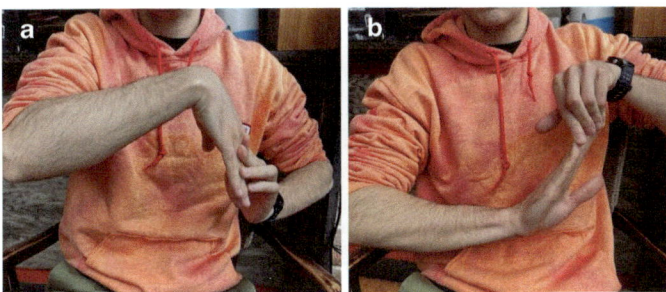

Fig. 9.3 (**a**, **b**) Maximal wrist passive flexion at 80° (**a**) and maximal wrist passive extension at 70° (**b**)

hand. Ask the patient to passively range all joints: the wrist, MCP, and IP joints, to the end range of flexion and extension (Fig. 9.3a, b) and the wrist into pronosupination and radial and ulnar deviation. A web-based goniometer can better estimate end flexion and extension of structures of interest.

Next, assess for active ROM abnormalities (Please see the Special Cases/Tests section, under Lacerations for a detailed description of this assessment, as it pertains to trauma).

Discriminating muscle strength is challenging via video without the provider's ability to apply graded resistance. The patient can demonstrate 3/5 resistance against gravity. Beyond this, one can grossly assess muscle strength greater than 3/5 by having the patient lift household items of increasing weight and relative to the opposite side.

Neurovascular Examination

Begin the vascular exam with a capillary refill test. Bring the fingernails into focus and inspect the fingernails and fingers for appropriate changes in color, or inappropriate discolorations. Subjective sensation is limited via video exam. The patient can follow the relevant anatomic sensory distribution with a chart online utilizing a paperclip or other sharp structure, as described by Van Nest et al. The easiest approach is to screenshare a sensory chart with the patient and systematically guide through hand distribution using the approach described below (Fig. 9.4a). Motor

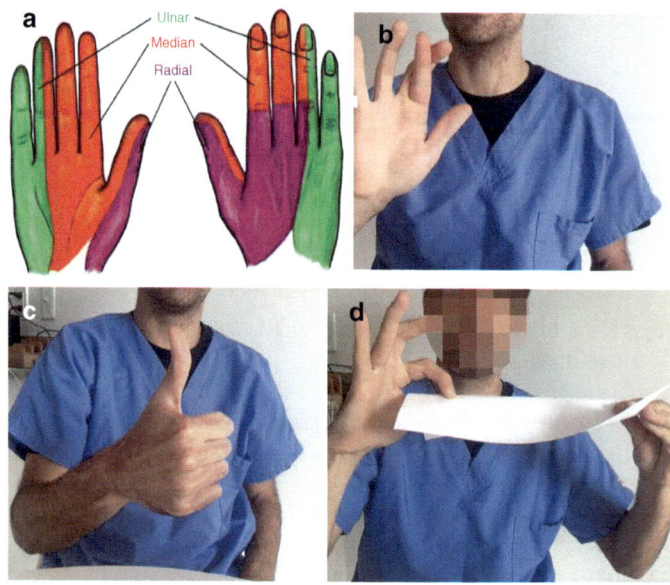

Fig. 9.4 (**a–d**) Sensory distribution and motor function ulnar, median, and radial nerves in the hand

function of the terminal median, radial, and ulnar branches are evaluated by maintenance of "OK sign"—thumb IP joint flexion from anterior interosseous nerve innervation of flexor pollicis longus. "Thumbs up sign"—thumb IP joint extension from posterior interosseous nerve of extensor pollicis longus, and "Crossed fingers"—interossei function from innervation by deep branch of ulnar nerve (Fig. 9.4b–d).

Differential Diagnosis

Scaphoid Fracture

The scaphoid carpal bone is a particularly important anatomical structure to palpate whenever there is a chief complaint of a fall on an outstretched hand, or a FOOSH injury. There are three

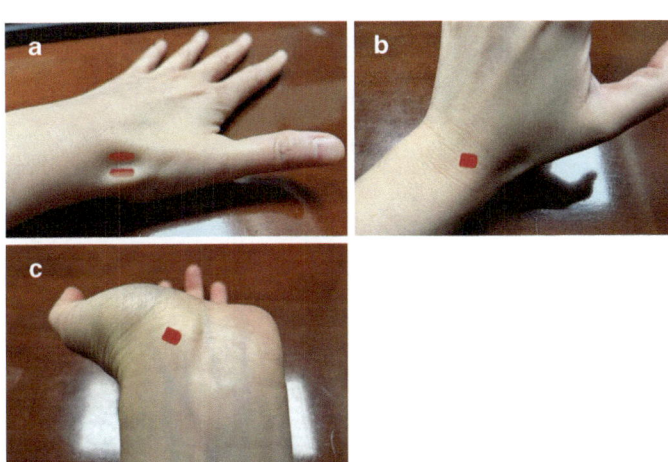

Fig. 9.5 (**a–c**) Scaphoid waist palpated at anatomic snuffbox (**a**), proximal scaphoid distal to Lister's tubercle (**b**), and distal scaphoid at palmar scaphoid tubercle (**c**)

places where the scaphoid can be palpated. These include: the scaphoid waist, the proximal scaphoid, and the distal scaphoid. The scaphoid waist is palpated at the anatomic snuffbox (Fig. 9.5a). The proximal edge of the scaphoid can be palpated distal to Lister's tubercle of the radius, on the dorsal side (Fig. 9.5b). And the distal scaphoid (scaphoid tubercle) can be palpated on the palmar side (Fig. 9.5c). Scaphoid fractures are important to identify due to their risk of avascular necrosis. Management of suspected scaphoid fractures are discussed further in the chapter.

Lacerations

In instances of trauma such as lacerations, it is particularly important to evaluate the function and active end ROM of all extrinsic and intrinsic hand muscles to confirm tendon and muscle integrity. Each flexor digitorum profundus is evaluated in isolation. The patient evaluates DIP flexion at the finger of interest by

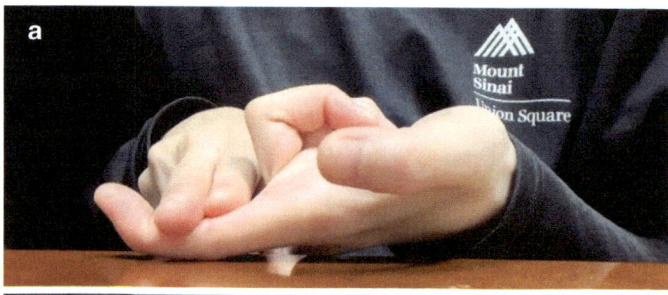

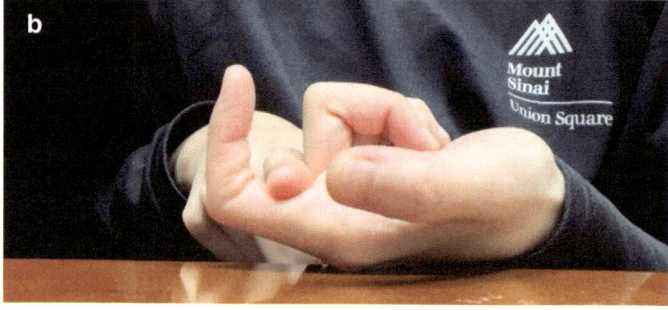

Fig. 9.6 (**a**, **b**) Flexion evaluation of FDP at DIP joint (**a**) and FDS at PIP joint (**b**)

immobilizing the PIP joint of that finger and the DIP joints of all remaining fingers (Fig. 9.6a). The patient is then asked to flex at the DIP and ROM is visualized. Each flexor digitorum superficialis is evaluated by asking the patient to flex at the PIP joint while the MCP joint of that finger and the PIP joints of all remaining fingers are held in immobilization (Fig. 9.6b).

Flexor pollicis longus is assessed with IP joint flexion while the MCP of the thumb is held in immobilization. Alternatively, the patient forms the "Okay sign," and active IP joint flexion is confirmed (Fig. 9.7).

To assess the extensor muscles of the hand and wrist, the patient places their hands flat on the table with palms faced down. In this position, the function and range of motion of the abductor pollicis longus and extensor pollicis brevis are evaluated with active abduction and extension, respectively, of the patient's

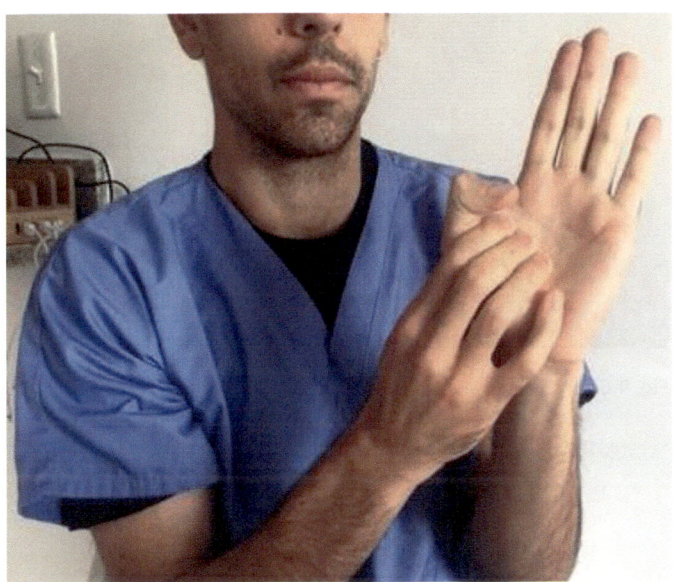

Fig. 9.7 Flexion evaluation of FPL at thumb IP joint

thumb. The patient actively lifts the thumb off the table surface to assess extensor pollicis longus function (Fig. 9.8).

To evaluate the extensor digitorum communis, the MCPs must be held in extension to eliminate the extensor contribution of the lumbricals. The patient hyperextends each digit independently off the table surface (Fig. 9.9).

Whenever a laceration is sustained to the dorsum of the PIP joint, concern should be raised for a central slip tendon injury. The extensor tendon of all digits trifurcates at the dorsal PIP joint, into the central slip and two lateral bands. All three structures extend the PIP joint. When the central slip is ruptured, PIP joint extension can be maintained by hyper-recruitment of the lateral bands. That hyper-recruitment is signified by the secondary function of the lateral bands—the taut, *hyperextension* of the DIP joint. A modified Elson's test can be performed to evaluate this injury [2]. In this test, the injured and contralateral fingers are abutted PIP to PIP at 90° flexion. The patient then extends DIPs. A normal test

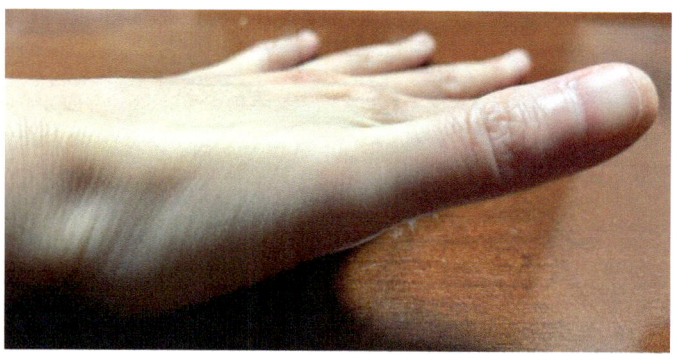

Fig. 9.8 Extension evaluation of EPL, "thumb off the table"

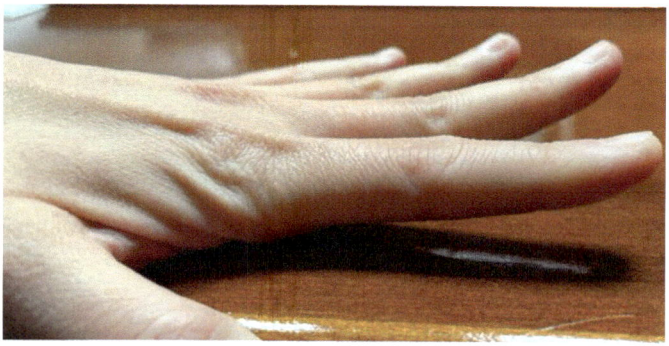

Fig. 9.9 Functional evaluation of EDC involves hyperextension of each finger off the table

shows symmetric extension of DIP. An injured central slip would manifest as asymmetric hyperextension at the DIP joint, suggesting a central slip injury (Fig. 9.10).

To evaluate the extensor muscles of the wrist, ask the patient to form a fist. The extensor carpi radialis brevis and longus are assessed with active extension and radial deviation of the wrist. The extensor carpi ulnaris is evaluated with active extension and ulnar deviation of the wrist. This completes the extrinsic hand muscle evaluation.

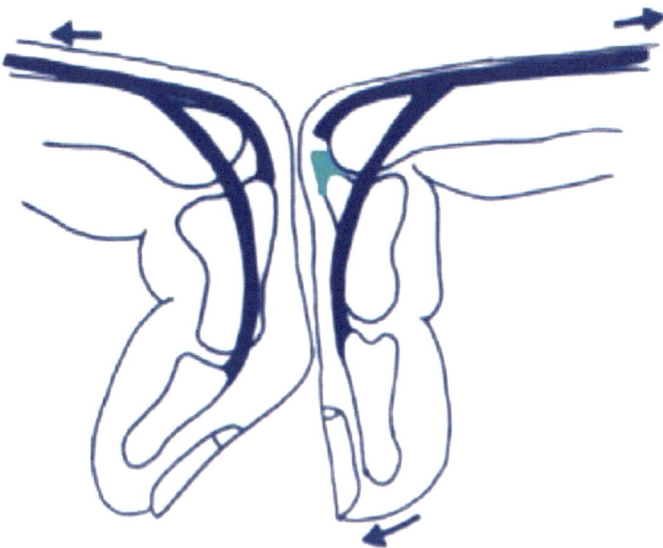

Fig. 9.10 Normal extensor mechanism involves central slip and two lateral bands trifurcating at the dorsal PIP joint. An injured central slip is revealed by an asymmetric hyperextension of the DIP joint, secondary to hyper-recruitment of the lateral bands

Evaluating the function and range of motion of the intrinsic muscles of the hand involves the lumbricals, interossei, and thenar muscles. The lumbricals are evaluated in sagittal view with MCP joint flexion and PIP joint extension (Fig. 9.11).

Interosseous muscle function is assessed by asking the patient to abduct, adduct, and cross their fingers. Lastly, the thenar muscles including opponens pollicis and hypothenar muscles are evaluated by opposition of the thumb and little finger, respectively.

Skier's/Gamekeeper's Thumb

Metacarpophalangeal ulnar ligament rupture (also referred to as Skier's, or Gamekeeper's, thumb) occurs when the ulnar collat-

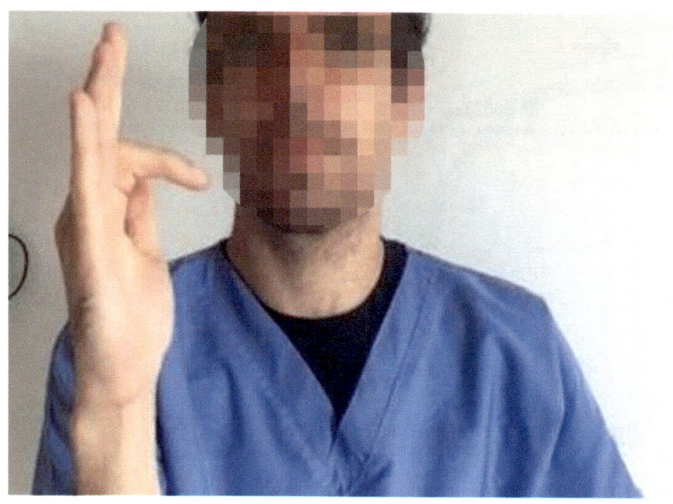

Fig. 9.11 Lumbrical function including MCP joint flexion and PIP joint extension

eral ligament of the first digit ruptures at the insertion into the proximal phalanx. The mechanism for this injury is radial deviation of the MCP, such as when a skier rapidly and forcefully decelerates with the hand gripping the ski poles (Fig. 9.12). Clinically, the patient will experience swelling and tenderness to palpation over ulnar border of the thumb MCP joint. They will also experience weakness to pincer grasp. To evaluate UCL tear, apply radial stress to the thumb with MCP held in both 30° and 0° degrees of flexion. A finding of >15° of laxity compared to the contralateral thumb, or 35° of total laxity, suggests a complete UCL rupture. XRs can show proximal phalanx volar subluxation as a finding suggestive of a UCL tear.

Jersey Finger

An avulsion, or tear, of the flexor tendon insertion from the distal phalanx of any digit is referred to as Jersey finger. The mechanism for this injury involves forced extension of a flexed DIP joint,

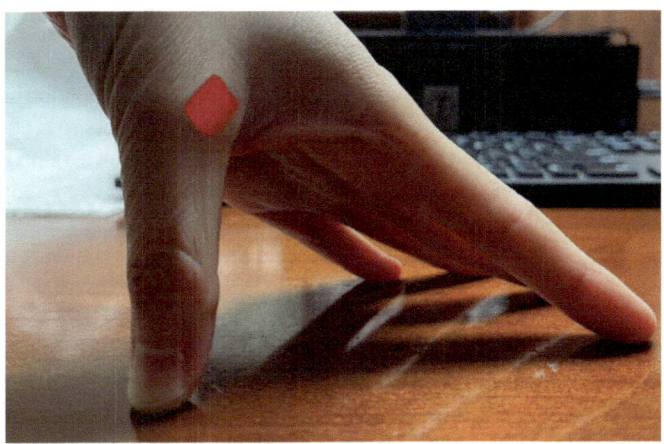

Fig. 9.12 The mechanism of UCL injury is radial deviation of thumb MCP joint

such as when a football player grabs onto a jersey of an opposing player with his fingertip. The diagnosis is clinical, with an inability to actively flex the DIP joint of the affected finger. Radiographs can show an accompanying volar avulsion fracture at the insertion point of the flexor tendon. Management of this injury is with full flexion immobilization of the DIP, PIP, MCP, and wrist joint with urgent follow-up, as nearly all these injuries are surgically managed and before significant retraction of the injured flexor tendon.

Mallet Finger

In contrast to Jersey Finger, Mallet finger involves a rupture of the extensor tendon distal to the DIP joint. It is caused by forced flexion of the extended DIP joint. The diagnosis is clinical, and the key finding is the DIP joint in passive resting flexion with the inability to actively extend the DIP. Radiography can show an accompanying dorsal avulsion fracture at the insertion point of the extensor tendon. Management involves splinting the DIP joint in hyperextension for 6 weeks. The PIP does not need to be additionally immobilized and is generally not advised.

De Quervain's Tenosynovitis

Inflammation of the synovial sheath that surrounds a tendon is termed tenosynovitis. De Quervain's tenosynovitis refers to tenosynovitis of the abductor pollicis longus (APL) and/or extensor pollicis brevis (EPB) tendons of the thumb, at the level where they pass adjacent to the styloid process of the radius. Risk factors include professions or hobbies that lead to overuse of the thumb, including "Blackberry's thumb." Mothers that frequently lift their infants are also at risk of developing "Toddler's thumb". Patients present with atraumatic pain at the radial side of the wrist made worse with thumb and wrist movements. On exam, there will be tenderness to palpation and swelling at the radial styloid at the first dorsal compartment, pain with abduction of the thumb, and decreased grip strength. Finkelstein test consists of the patient tucking a flexed thumb and placing the wrist into passive ulnar deviation to eccentrically stretch the affected tendons. Pain with this test indicates a positive Finkelstein test. Same-day treatment often includes brief thumb spica immobilization.

Flexor Tenosynovitis

Most cases of infectious tenosynovitis occur in the upper extremities, and more often in the flexor sheaths rather than the extensor sheaths of tendons. Suspicion should be raised when there is a history of a bite, recent surgery, or an open injury. Kanavel signs are the four cardinal signs of flexor tenosynovitis that help establish the diagnosis, and include: tenderness along the course of the flexor sheath, symmetric or fusiform enlargement of the affected digit, the affected finger held in passive flexion, and pain along the tendon with passive extension. These signs have a high sensitivity but low specificity, with the earliest sign being pain with passive extension. The differential diagnosis includes gout, HSV infection, rheumatoid arthritis, and inflammation from local trauma. The definitive diagnosis is made with tendon sheath aspiration and cultures. The treatment mainstay is surgical washout. For cases with early presentation, a trial of antibiotics can be acceptable, with close inpatient monitoring for progression of symptoms.

Carpal Tunnel Syndrome

Repetitive wrist flexion and extension can lead to inflammation and compression of the median nerve at the carpal tunnel. This leads to a median nerve mononeuropathy. Risk factors for carpal tunnel syndrome include hypothyroidism, rheumatoid arthritis, diabetes mellitus, obesity, female sex, and pregnancy. Signs include pain, paresthesias, and numbness in the median nerve distribution which includes the palmar sides of the first three digits of the hand, and the radial side of the fourth digit. Patients often awaken at night with burning pain and tingling of the hand. Abnormal sensation of the distal palmar tip of the second digit is the most sensitive sign, whereas decreased sensation in the radial side of the fourth digit relative to the ulnar side is the most specific.

There are various diagnostic maneuvers and tests described. The Phalen test and Tinel sign are the two classic maneuvers; however, both suffer from poor sensitivity and specificity. The Phalen test involves holding the wrists in flexion against each other for 60 s. Tinel sign involves percussing the palmar aspect of the wrist. The Durkan sign, also known as the carpal compression test, involves compressing the carpal tunnel for 30 s. The Hand Elevation test has recently been found to be the most sensitive and specific. The patient raises both arms above their head for 2 min. A positive test of all the above tests involves a reproduction or exacerbation of the patient's symptoms [3].

Special Considerations

- Given the high functionality and vulnerabilities of our hand and wrist, soft tissue injuries can be as consequential as osseous. The subtlety between benign versus high morbidity injuries is challenging to discern virtually.
- Proper immobilization can be more time sensitive than arriving at a definitive diagnosis. Implement a very low threshold for empiric immobilization to prevent progression of symptoms and instability. The tradeoff risk of joint stiffness and muscle atrophy is much less than in medium to larger joints. Radiology

and DME/bracing can typically be coordinated as outpatient referrals.
- Activity restrictions including in weight bearing activities, contact or collision sports, and occupational demands should be recommended and quantified.

Management/Treatment

A FOOSH injury is a common mechanism for which a range of pathology can result, affecting any part of the upper extremity. The telemedicine visit should begin with a triage process to determine which patients should be immediately referred to the ED, and which can be safely managed as outpatient.

Any patient presenting with an open deformity, visible deformity, or vascular compromise from the shoulder to the distal hand requires prompt ED referral. The inspection and range of motion of the physical exam are key parameters in this process of ruling-out emergent injuries, whereas special tests are focused on diagnostic "rule-in's."

For a closed wrist injury with a reassuring neurovascular exam, a trial of PRICE (protected weight bearing, rest, ice, compression, elevation) can be initiated. The typical mainstay for a FOOSH injury may be a removable volar wrist splint or thumb spica splint, if radial sided structures are implied. These can be purchased from a nearby pharmacy or surgical supply store, or a DME group can be contracted to provide in-home orthotics. Non-weight bearing or partial weight bearing as guided by symptoms, and non-contact activities is recommended and documented. Anti-inflammatory agents are recommended ranging from topical ice and thermal therapies, topical NSAID's, and oral NSAID's of varying grades. Elevation of the affected limb is recommended, especially when sedentary or nocturnal. The hand and wrist offer a strong vascular supply in tight compartments, and marked swelling can rapidly develop.

The timing of outpatient imaging and follow-up appointment varies by the differential diagnosis. Outpatient radiology includes radiograph, ultrasound, or MRI and can often be coordinated during this interval. Given the subtleties of hand and wrist injuries, a subsequent on-site visit is typically recommended for a direct exam. Injuries that may require a procedural intervention can be arranged for advanced testing or virtual consultations on an expedited timeline. Injuries that may resolve with conservative strategies can be evaluated in 7–10 days, as serial physical exams and radiographs can provide more valuable information after a short and necessary period of PRICE.

Complications/Red Flags: Potential Limb Threatening Conditions Requiring Emergent Intervention

- **Compartment syndrome**—common with crush injury caused by compression of hand/wrist neurovascular structures from severe muscle swelling. The most commonly involved compartments are dorsal and palmar interossei, the thenar and hypothenar, the adductor, and individual fingers. Clinical diagnosis involves pain out of proportion to exam with tense swelling in the affected compartment. Pain is classically deep and poorly localized but replicated with passive stretch of the involved compartment muscles.
- **High pressure injection injury**—occurs as an occupational injury using high pressure spray tools for paint, grease, solvents, and oil. The injections from these tools can occur at forces of 3000–10,000 PSU (400 mph), and even small volumes of injectant can cause catastrophic sequelae such as compartment syndrome. It commonly occurs in the non-dominant hand or finger. It is important to clarify what type of material was injected as water-based materials are far less toxic than grease-based ones. Always examine far distal to the site of injection as the fragments can track through fascial planes of least resistance.
- **Open fracture**—is defined as a fracture that communicates with the outside environment. The fracture portion does not

have to be overtly exposed and can be smaller than anticipated, so treat as an open fracture regardless of how small the overlying wound is. Graded based on the Gustilo–Anderson scale, grade III injuries involve the neurovascular structures while grade 1 fractures are not overly contaminated and lack extensive soft tissue damage [4].
- **Amputation**—If the amputated finger is available, prepare with irrigation and wrap in moist sterile gauze. Pug it into a plastic bag and place the bag in ice water, avoiding direct exposure to ice. Chilling may keep the digit viable for 24 h versus 12 h. Classically, if the amputation is distal to the DIP, the patient is not a candidate for reimplantation.
- **Vascular injury**—Every patient should be evaluated for hard signs of vascular injury that demand immediate arterial exploration. These include: absent distal pulses, signs of distal ischemia (6 Ps: pain, pallor, paresthesia, paralysis, poikilothermia, pulselessness), audible bruit or palpable thrill, active pulsatile hemorrhage, or large expanding hematoma. Soft signs may present on telemedicine that must be referred for advanced managing including: non-expanding hematoma, subjectively decreased pulse, peripheral nerve deficit, history of pulsatile or significant hemorrhage at the time of injury, unexplained hypotension, or high-risk orthopedic injuries (fracture, dislocation, penetration).
- **Burns—thermal, chemical** are classified as superficial, superficial partial, deep partial, full, or fourth degree depending on the deepest skin structure involved and the appearance of the burn. In an electrical burn, the primary determinant of injury is the amount of current delivered, and AC injuries are classically worse than DC as it is difficult to release the affected extremity from the electric source. Review local burn unit criteria for indications to refer for advanced management, where hand and wrist involvement is typically an indication for emergent transfer.

Follow-Up

Musculoskeletal injuries are managed by a wide variety of medical and surgical specialties, with the work of allied health specialties including physical, occupational, and hand therapies, nutrition, ergonomics, orthotics, exercise science, and social work. Many of these services have developed telemedicine models for successful coordination and delivery of virtual care.

References

1. Van Nest BA, et al. Telemedicine evaluation and techniques in hand surgery. J Hand Surg Glob Online. 2020;2(4):240–5.
2. Schreuders TA, Soeters JN, Hovius SE. A modification of Elson's test for the diagnosis of an acute extensor central slip injury. Br J Hand Ther. 2006;11(4):111–2.
3. Singh V, Ericson WB Jr. Median nerve entrapments in peripheral nerve entrapments. Cham: Springer International Publishing; 2016. p. 369–82.
4. Kim PH, Leopold SS. Gustilo–Anderson classification. Clin Orthop Relat Res. 2012;470(11):3270–4.

The Telemedicine Hip Exam

Jasmin Harounian, Carley Trentman, and Richard G. Chang

In this chapter, we will be discussing how to conduct a telemedicine visit when there is a concern of an underlying hip or pelvic etiology. The chapter will be broken down by chief complaint, the proper physical exam techniques, creating an effective differential, special considerations, management, and treatment, as well as complications and red flags.

Chief Complaint/Patient History

The purpose of obtaining a patient history is multi-fold: It should rule out any concerning sources of hip pathology such as malignancy, infection, or systemic disease; further differentiate hip pain from back pain; and narrow down an otherwise broad differential to enable performing a focused physical exam [1]. As with any musculoskeletal injury, mechanism of injury and any attempted treatment modalities should be ascertained. If pain is the chief complaint, ask the patient to further characterize the location and radiation pattern, severity, quality, onset, and duration, as well as any alleviating or aggravating factors. Mechanical symptoms

J. Harounian (✉) · C. Trentman · R. G. Chang
Department of Rehabilitation and Human Performance, Icahn School of Medicine at Mount Sinai, New York, NY, USA
e-mail: richard.chang@mountsinai.org

© The Author(s), under exclusive license to Springer Nature Switzerland AG 2023
M. Zakhary et al. (eds.), *Telemedicine for the Musculoskeletal Physical Exam*, https://doi.org/10.1007/978-3-031-16873-4_10

such as snapping, popping, locking, clicking, and subjective instability should also be elicited. Pain or catching during flexion and axial loading activities such as rising from a seated position, walking up or down stairs, or entering and exiting a vehicle can also imply mechanical hip pain [2]. A history of acute onset or trauma is a better prognostic indicator than an insidious onset of symptoms [3]. A history of acute onset or trauma is a better prognostic indicator than an insidious onset of symptoms [4].

Physical Exam

Setup

Prior to beginning the virtual hip examination, ensure that the patient's environment has adequate lighting. Looser fitting pants, such as athletic shorts, are preferred for this portion of the examination. If the patient is comfortable with a significant other, friend, or family member holding the camera, this may be the most optimal for properly conducting the telemedicine visit.

Inspection

Have the patient rise from a seated to standing position. Note any difficulty the patient may have with this transfer. If possible, have the camera scan the entire anterior and posterior surfaces of the lower legs, taking note of any areas of erythema, ecchymosis, scarring, or deformity. Note any external rotation of the ankle (this could be indicative of femoral retroversion), or excessive internal rotation (potentially indicative of femoral anteversion). Note if the patient is standing with either knee in a flexed position to potentially offload the involved limb. Knee alignment may be assessed here as well, with genu varum or genu valgum identified. Also look for any asymmetry of the shoulders, torso or hips which could indicate a component of scoliosis or a leg length discrepancy [5]. If there is any concern for asymmetry in thigh circumference which can be seen with a femoral neuropathy, have the patient use measuring tape to measure the widest circumference of each thigh. Have the patient turn to have their side facing the camera in order to assess for posterior pelvic tilt which results in a flat back, or anterior pelvic tilt—which can appear as excessive lumbar lordosis or a curved back [1].

Gait

Now that the patient is standing, assess the patient's gait. There should be enough room to permit a full-body view of walking both toward and away from the camera. Assess for any circumduction, excessive trunk extension, or instability. To assess for hip abductor pathology (affecting gluteus medius and minimus tendons), look for a Trendelenburg sign. Prior to checking this, ensure the patient has a place of support (e.g., nearby wall or chair) and a flat surface to stand on in order to prevent any risk for falls. Ask the patient to stand with their backs facing the camera with their hands on their hips. Then, ask the patient to stand on the contralateral leg, taking note of any ipsilateral drop in hip height with the stance leg.

Range of Motion

For each movement, start with the unaffected side in order to compare any differences in range of motion.

Hip Flexion
With the patient lying supine, ask the patient to bring the knee in toward their chest as far as they can.

Hip Abduction
Ask the patient to slide their leg out to the side.

Hip Adduction
Ask the patient to lift the other leg and slide the leg being tested in toward midline and under the lifted leg.

Internal Rotation

Ask the patient to flex the hip to 90° and move the heel out to the side as far as they can.

External Rotation

Ask the patient to flex the hip to 90° and move the heel inwards as far as they can.

Palpation

Next, instruct the patient to point to the area in question with one finger. Guide the patient through both light and deep palpation of the area in question. Then, guide the patient through palpation of the greater trochanter. Ask the patient to lay on their asymptomatic side and face the camera. Have the patient flex their hips to roughly 60° with their knees together [2]. Then, ask the patient to palpate the lateral hip to assess for any tenderness along the greater trochanter.

Muscle Testing

Have the patient rise from a seated to standing position. Note any difficulty the patient may have with this transfer. Ask the patient to perform both a double-legged and single-legged squat while facing the camera and note any weakness, dynamic knee valgus, or difficulty with this maneuver. The patient can hold onto a sturdy object such as a chair or table for the single-legged squat if there is concern for issues with balance. Have the patient take several steps on their heels as well as their toes to assess for any foot drop.

If there is an assistant helping the patient during the visit, ask them to help perform manual muscle testing with the patient seated. For hip flexion, ask the patient to lift their knee and maintain its elevation against resistance. For knee extension, ask the patient to straighten their leg while the assistant is holding the patient's knee with one hand and applying resistance against the distal leg with the other hand. For ankle dorsiflexion, ask the patient to bring their ankle and toes up toward the ceiling while having the assistant provide downward resistance. For extensor hallucis longus extension, ask the patient to lift their big toe up toward the ceiling while having the assistant provide downward resistance. Lastly, for ankle plantar flexion, ask the patient to press downward with their ankle against resistance from the assistant, as though they are pressing a gas pedal. Note any asymmetry in strength between the affected and unaffected side.

Sensation

Have the patient lightly touch along the anterior, lateral, and posterior thighs and assess for any difference in sensation, paresthesias, or numbness. If the patient has a cotton ball and a safety pin available, these objects can be used to test for light touch and pinprick, respectively.

Special Tests

Modified Log Roll
With the patient lying supine on a bed or couch and their camera propped on a chair or held by an assistant, have the patient start with the unaffected side and actively roll their leg in and out. Note any discomfort or asymmetry in range as compared to the unaffected side.

FABER (Flexion, ABduction, External Rotation of the Hip)
With the patient lying supine on a bed or couch and their camera propped on a chair or held by an assistant, ask the patient to make a figure 4 position with their leg—effectively flexing the hip and abducting/externally rotating the leg. Then ask the patient to apply pressure to the medial surface of the flexed knee, noting if this elicits any pain in the ipsilateral hip or contralateral SI joint.

Modified Stinchfield

If there is concern for hip flexor pathology, the patient can perform the Modified Stinchfield test or Active Straight Leg Raise. With the patient lying supine on a bed or couch and their camera propped on a chair or held by an assistant, have the patient flex the affected hip while maintaining a straight leg. Then, ask the patient to apply downward pressure above the knee of the affected leg. Note any pain along the iliopsoas muscle or groin.

Sit-Up or Resisted Sit-Up

If there is concern for a sports hernia, core muscle injury, or athletic pubalgia, the patient can be asked to perform a sit-up or a resisted sit-up. Have the patient lying supine with the camera positioned appropriately. With their knees bent and feet planted on the ground, ask the patient to perform a regular sit-up. If there is an assistant available, they can be asked to provide resistance against the patient's chest or shoulders during the sit-up. The test is positive if the patient reports reproduction of symptoms in the groin with the increase in abdominal pressure during the sit-up.

Seated Slump Test/Straight Leg Raise

If there is concern for radicular pain originating from the lumbar spine, the patient can perform a seated slump test and/or a seated straight leg raise. For the seated slump test, the patient should be in a seated position facing the camera. Ask the patient to slump forward with their upper torso flexed forward. Next, ask the patient to bring their chin to their chest and extend the knee of the affected leg. Finally, ask the patient to dorsiflex their foot, bringing their toes toward their nose and effectively increasing any neural tension. A positive test would entail any reproduction of neurological symptoms such as radiating, sharp, shooting pain into the leg. See the lumbar spine chapter for further exam maneuvers dedicated to lumbar spine pathology.

Resisted Hip Adduction

If there is concern for an adductor muscle strain, the patient can be asked to perform resisted hip adduction. Have the patient seated and facing the camera with their feet planted on the floor. Ask the patient to make two fists and place them in tandem between their knees. Then, have the patient adduct their hips by squeezing their legs inwards against their fists. The test is positive if this reproduces pain along the inner thigh.

Single Leg Hop Test

If there is concern for a stress fracture, the patient can be asked to perform the single leg hop test. Ask the patient to stand on the affected leg and hop up and down on that foot. The test is positive if the patient reports localization and reproduction of their pain with hopping.

Differential Diagnosis

Due to the broad nature of the category, the differential diagnosis with respect to various pathologies involving the hip has been delineated in the chart below [1].

Soft tissue injuries	Bone injuries	Nerve entrapment injuries	Intra-articular pathology
Bursopathies/bursitis (trochanteric, ischial, iliopsoas, iliopectineal)	Degenerative joint disease of the hip	Sciatic nerve entrapment	Labral tears
Contusions (iliac crest, quadriceps, groin)	Traumatic fractures	Obturator nerve entrapment	Femoral acetabular impingement (FAI)
Strains and/or tendinopathies (core muscle injury/athletic pubalgia, adductor, iliopsoas, external oblique, hamstring, quadriceps)	Stress fractures (pelvic, sacral, femoral neck)	Pudendal nerve entrapment	Loose bodies

Soft tissue injuries	Bone injuries	Nerve entrapment injuries	Intra-articular pathology
Hernias (inguinal, femoral)	Osteitis pubis	Ilioinguinal nerve entrapment	Chondral injuries
	Osteonecrosis	Femoral nerve entrapment	Septic arthritis
	SI joint dysfunction	Lateral femoral cutaneous nerve entrapment (meralgia paresthetica)	
	Lumbar spine pathology		

Special Considerations

For the pediatric population, other diagnoses to consider include developmental hip dysplasia, avulsion fractures, slipped capital femoral epiphysis, and Legg–Calve–Perthes disease. Additionally, beware of non-musculoskeletal causes that can also mimic intra-articular or extra-articular hip pain. These can include bony malignancies or tumors in the pelvis or hip; systemic inflammatory conditions such as rheumatoid arthritis affecting the hip joint; or genitourinary conditions like sexually transmitted diseases, which can cause groin lymphadenopathy.

Management/Treatment

- Soft tissues injuries such as bursitis/bursopathies, contusions, acute muscle strains, and/or tendinopathies can often be treated with conservative at home management. This entails a combination of activity modification, physical therapy, and a home exercise program. If there is concern for an inguinal hernia, this would require referral to another specialty provider (e.g., general surgery) for further evaluation. If there is any concern of an incarcerated or strangulated hernia, this would require referral for more urgent management.

- Bone injuries can range from fractures to osteoarthritis. Stress fractures, traumatic fractures, and hip osteonecrosis should be referred to an orthopedist for surgical evaluation once imaging is obtained. Osteoarthritis, osteitis pubis, SI joint dysfunction, and lumbar spine pathology can often be treated initially with conservation management. This entails a combination of activity modification, physical therapy, and a home exercise program.
- Nerve entrapment injuries may require an electromyography test with nerve conduction studies to differentiate peripheral nerve injuries from a lumbosacral plexopathy or radiculopathy.
- Intra-articular hip pathologies such as labral tears, femoral acetabular impingement, loose bodies, and chondral injuries often require imaging studies to evaluate the full extent of injury. If surgical intervention is needed, the patient should be referred to an orthopedist for this evaluation. If septic arthritis is suspected, the patient should present to the nearest ED for emergent evaluation as this is an orthopedic emergency.

Complications/Red Flags

- If there are any signs of fever, chills, malaise, night sweats, or unintended weight loss upon review of systems and/or if there is any significant swelling, erythema upon inspection of the area in question, this should warrant further investigation with an in-person visit for an underlying malignancy or infection.
- If there is a history of trauma to the affected side, this should warrant imaging studies of the bilateral hips in order to have a comparison view of the unaffected side. The patient should present to the nearest Emergency Department for further evaluation following a trauma to ensure no other injuries were incurred.
- If there is concern for a septic hip joint, the patient should be instructed to present to the nearest Emergency Department for further evaluation as this is an orthopedic emergency.

References

1. Miller MD, Thompson SR. DeLee & Drez's orthopaedic sports medicine E-book. Amsterdam: Elsevier Health Sciences; 2018.
2. O'Leary JA, Berend K, Vail TP. The relationship between diagnosis and outcome in arthroscopy of the hip. Arthroscopy. 2001;17:181–8.
3. Byrd JW, Jones KS. Prospective analysis of hip arthroscopy with 2-year follow-up. Arthroscopy. 2000;16:578–87.
4. Malanga GA, Mautner K. Musculoskeletal physical examination: an evidence-based approach, vol. 8. 2nd ed. Amsterdam: Elsevier; 2016. p. 145–72.
5. Laskowski ER, Johnson SE, Shelerud RA, et al. The telemedicine musculoskeletal examination. Mayo Clin Proc. 2020;95(8):1715–31.

The Telemedicine Knee Exam

11

Michelle N. Leong, Laurenie G. Louissaint, and Joseph Herrera

History

Like all clinical encounters, the first step is to obtain a thorough history. Detailed questions are important to filter through your differential diagnoses, especially since this is not a hands-on visit. Typical questions:

- Chief complaint
- Onset
- Inciting event: if so, specific mechanism of injury
- Location: Have patient point to area(s) of pain
- Duration

M. N. Leong (✉) · L. G. Louissaint · J. Herrera
Department of Rehabilitation and Human Performance, Icahn School of Medicine, Mount Sinai Hospital, New York, NY, USA
e-mail: michelle.leong@mountsinai.org;
laurenie.louissaint@mountsinai.org; joseph.herrera@mountsinai.org

© The Author(s), under exclusive license to Springer Nature Switzerland AG 2023
M. Zakhary et al. (eds.), *Telemedicine for the Musculoskeletal Physical Exam*, https://doi.org/10.1007/978-3-031-16873-4_11

- Exacerbating factors
- Relieving factors
- Radiation of pain
- Associated symptoms: redness, swelling, sensory changes
- Severity
- Review of systems: fever, chills, chest pain, shortness of breath, urinary symptoms, diarrhea, rash, etc.
- Treatments tried

Obtain details on past medical history, past surgical history, family history, allergies, and social history.

Physical Exam

To begin the physical exam, patients should be located in an uncluttered room with bright light. Proper lower body clothing includes shorts, no socks, and no shoes. In an ideal setting, the patient would have a second person available to assist with the physical exam.

Two Person Physical Exam

Inspection and Gait
Have the assistant hold the camera so the patient is in full view as they move from a seated to standing position. Have the assistant adjust so the full body is in view. While the patient is facing the camera, have the patient lift up the shorts to view for any asymmetry or atrophy. Have them stand straight, ankles together to inspect for deformities or genu valgum/varus. Have them turn to the sides and inspect. Then, ask the patient to walk up and down a long hallway, if possible. If not, the length of the room a few times should suffice. Be sure to have adequate viewing time of the patient walking facing the camera and facing away from the camera.

Before the patient lies down, have the assistant bring the camera to the back of the knees for inspection of the popliteal fossa, hamstring muscles, and calf muscles. Next, have the patient lie down on a sofa. Ask the assistant to move the mobile device closer to the patient's affected knee(s) to start off with visual inspection. Once inspection of the affected knee(s) is complete, ask the assistant to step back in order to view both knees at once to compare. Depending on camera quality, providers may need to confirm with the assistant whether the area is erythematous.

Range of Motion Testing

Next, have the assistant prop the mobile device in horizontal position at around or higher than coffee table height. Help them adjust the camera position so you are able to see the full lower half of the body. To prevent extra positional changes, have the affected side near the edge of the sofa. Have the assistant go through passive range of motion (ROM) by taking the non-affected leg and bending at the hips. First, can check for full flexion of the hip (Bend the knee as close to the chest as possible), external rotation (place them in a Fig. 11.4), and internal rotation (place them in a reverse Fig. 11.4). Once the hip has been checked, ask the assistant to place the patient's foot flat on the sofa and bend the knee as much as possible to double check the range of knee flexion (web-based goniometer?). Then, ask the assistant to straighten the leg out to test knee extension. While the leg is in motion, ask if the assistant can hear any crackling or crunching sounds. Also have the assistant place a hand over the kneecap to palpate for any crepitus during ROM. Do the same steps as above on the affected side. Throughout the ROM testing, determine if there is any pain with ROM.

Palpation

Have the assistant palpate for warmth (place your palms on the patient's knees; does one feel warmer?) Using firm pressure, the assistant can palpate around both patellas to determine if one knee has more fluid than another, suggesting effusion. Also have them compare any prominences to determine if equal on both sides, or if the mass is soft and moveable, or hard and bony. Have them find the "dents" to the sides of the middle of the patella to locate the joint lines. Have them use their thumbs to palpate the joint lines one at a time and determine if the patient has any pain in a particular area. Then have the assistant palpate beneath the patella for the patellar tendon, medially for medial collateral ligament, laterally for lateral collateral ligament, and inferiorly and medially for pes anserine bursa. Complete palpation for both knees.

Strength Testing

Start off with the camera directly facing the patient, standing propped up on a table, so the lower half of the body can be seen while the patient is sitting. Ask the assistant to sit on a chair to the side while strength testing the patient to avoid blocking the camera, while also protecting their own body mechanics. While the patient is sitting, have the patient hold up one leg as if marching while the assistant resists the effort. Ask the patient to nearly straighten their leg completely while the assistant attempts to bend the knee. Ask the patient to bend their ankle up and back while the assistant resists. Ask the patient to lift the big toe up while the assistant resists. Ask the patient to push their foot against the assistant's hand like pushing on a gas pedal. For each test, compare each side before moving onto the next area. Also, ask the assistant if the resistance was full strength, some strength, only able to lift against gravity, or unable to lift against gravity. Physicians should also feel free to perform the desired motion to guide both the patient and the assistant. Providing verbal cues such as "toes to nose" or "press the gas pedal" may help patients understand the movement that needs to be performed.

Sensation Testing

Ask the assistant to lightly touch the upper thighs, lower thighs, inner shin, side of shin, top of foot, bottom of foot, on both sides at the same time to compare light touch sensation. To test pin prick sensation, ask the assistant to use a safety pin's sharp point in the same areas.

Reflex Testing

To test patellar reflexes, have a small hand/face towel available. Have the assistant feel for the bottom edge of the patella. Move slightly beneath the bony edge. Ask the assistant to use the edge of a smartphone or television remote to lightly tap beneath the kneecap. Use the small towel folded in half for a thin cushion as necessary. Test both sides. To test Achilles reflex, have the assistant feel for the Achilles tendon above the heel bone. Ask the assistant to bend the ankle up slightly and lightly tap on the tendon with the smartphone or television remote. Test both sides.

Provocative Testing [1]

Supine Provocative Testing

Patellar Apprehension
With the patient relaxed and with a slight bend to the knee, push on the medial (inner side) of the kneecap laterally (towards the outer side). If the patient becomes apprehensive and uncomfortable the more laterally the patella is placed, or tries to straighten the knee, this is considered positive.

Patellar Compression Test (Clarke Sign)
Knee is fully extended. Have the assistant place their thumb and forefinger at the top of the patella and push down into the sofa and towards the feet. Have the patient attempt to straighten out their knee more (contracting the quadriceps muscles). Pain would suggest patellofemoral dysfunction.

Anterior and Posterior Drawer
Have the assistant flex the hip "halfway" (about 45°). Have the assistant place a knee or sit on the patient's foot. Advise the assistant to hold the leg at the top of the shin with both hands, fingers around calf muscle and thumbs along the bone and near the bottom of the kneecap. Have the assistant pull the shin towards them and away from them, noting if it feels "loose." Complete and compare both sides.

McMurray
Have the assistant fully flex the hip and knee. Place one hand on the knee with fingers along the "dents" or joint lines of the knee.

The other hand will be holding the heel/foot. Internally rotate (twist the lower leg towards the middle or inside) and straighten the knee. Feel for any clicking or patient sensation of knee giving way. Repeat but have the assistant externally rotate (twist the lower leg towards the outside or laterally) and straighten the knee.

Prone Provocative Testing
Ask the patient to lie on their stomach, if able.

Apley Grind Test
Have the patient bend their knee to 90° (L-shaped). Have the assistant grab the foot in both hands. The assistant should place a downward pressure on the foot down towards the sofa while twisting the foot and lower leg. Have the patient vocalize and localize pain.

Seated Provocative Testing
While seated and prior to provocative testing, the assistant can wrap both hands around the knee, using fingers to feel the back of the knee for any masses.

Varus Stress Test
Have the assistant place one hand in the medial (inside) knee and the ankle. While placing pressure on the inside of the knee, bring the ankle medially (towards the middle of the body.) Ask the patient if the motion causes pain, or if the assistant can feel one side separating more than the other.

Valgus Stress Test
Have the assistant place one hand in the lateral (outside) knee and the ankle. While placing pressure on the outside of the knee, bring the ankle laterally (away from the middle of the body). Ask the patient if the motion causes pain, or if the assistant can feel one side separating more than the other.

Standing Provocative Testing

Two-Legged Squat
Have the patient hold onto a table or the assistant. With feet flat on the ground and about shoulder-width apart, have them bend at the knees and squat down. Have the patient vocalize and localize any pain. Monitor for ability and instability.

Duck Walk (Childress Test)
While fully squatting down, have the patient try and walk forward, backward, sideways. The patient can hold onto the assistant or furniture if needed. Have the patient vocalize and localize any pain or clicking, or the inability to stay in the squat position.

One-Legged Squat
While holding onto the assistant or furniture, have the patient squat on one leg. Attempt on both sides. Have the patient vocalize and localize any pain and note any inability to complete the motion due to instability or weakness.

Thessaly Test
While holding onto the assistant or furniture, have the patient stand on one leg with foot flat on the ground and knee slightly bent. Ask them to rotate their body to twist around the knee. Have the patient vocalize and localize the pain. Repeat on the other side.

One Person Examination

Inspection and Gait
After the history interview, ask the patient to hold their phone and "flip" the camera so it is not in "selfie" mode. Have the patient sit at the edge of the seat, straighten their knees while sitting down (keeping the legs relaxed with heels touching the ground) and point the camera so both knees are in view. Compare and inspect the anterior knees. Then have the patient point the camera at the

unaffected side, then to the affected side for inspection. Depending on camera quality, providers may need to clarify if there is any erythema.

Ask the patient to prop the camera standing up on a desk height table. Scoot the chair far enough back so the camera has a good view of the full body. Ask the patient to move from a sitting to standing position. While the patient is facing the camera, have the patient lift up the shorts to view for any asymmetry or atrophy. Have them stand straight, ankles together to inspect for deformities or genu valgum/varus. Have them turn to the side and inspect. Have the patient walk as far away as possible from the camera and towards the camera multiple times to observe gait. Have the patient turn away from the camera and have them adjust themselves so the back of the legs are in view of the camera for inspection.

Range of Motion Testing

Have the patient move the camera to about coffee table height and prop the camera standing up. Ideally, the patient would have an armless chair. Position the chair so that the camera can view the lower half of the body easily.

Have the patient sit back down. Have the patient pivot in the chair so the camera is facing their lateral side. If the patient is facing the right side, have them flex (bend) their left knee (Fig. 11.1) as much as possible while their left palm is located on the patella to feel for crepitus (crunching). An online goniometer may be used for accurate degrees of range. Then have the patient extend (straighten) their knee as much as possible (Fig. 11.2). Have them pivot in the chair so the camera is now looking at the other side. Complete the same steps. While seated, ask the patient to place their lateral ankle on the other thigh in a Fig. 11.4 position to test external rotation of the hip. Compare both sides. To test internal rotation, ask the patient to place one knee on top of the other with the heel facing outward. Compare both sides. The patient can also use a towel beneath the foot and held in both hands to help externally rotate and internally rotate (Figs. 11.3 and 11.4).

11 The Telemedicine Knee Exam

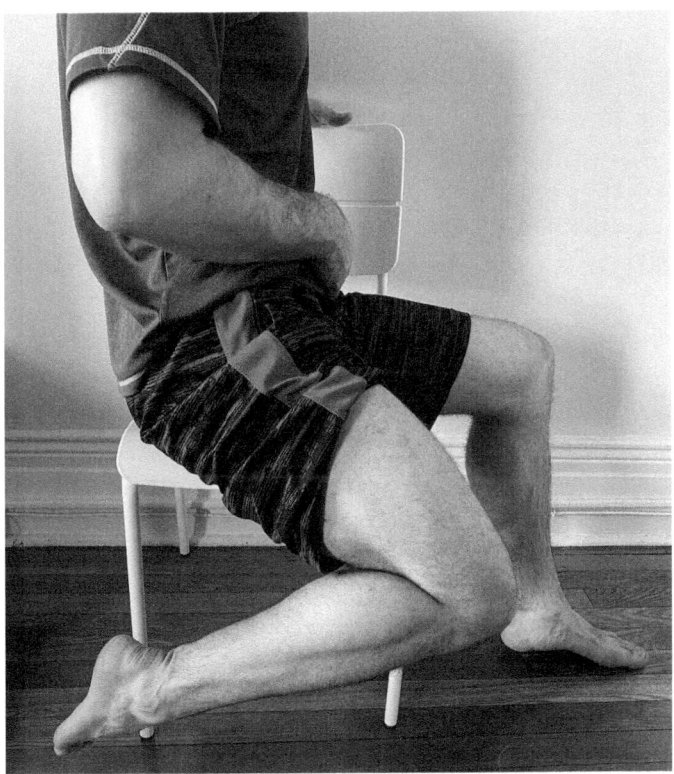

Fig. 11.1 Seated active knee flexion ROM testing

Palpation

Have the patient place their hands on their knees, noticing for any warmth, size difference, or fluid compared to the other. Then, have the patient palpate the unaffected side first. Using firm pressure, the patient can palpate around each patella to determine if one knee has more fluid than another. While palpating each patella, have the patient compare any prominences to determine if equal on both sides, or if the mass is soft and moveable, or hard and bony. Have the patient find the "dents" to the sides of the

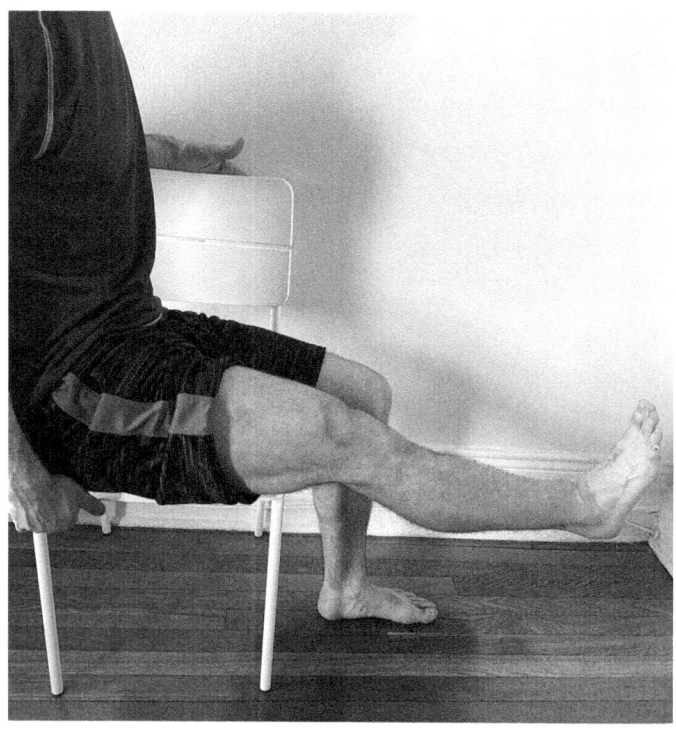

Fig. 11.2 Seated active knee extension ROM testing

middle of the patella to locate the joint lines. Have the patient use their thumb to push along the medial, then lateral joint lines, one at a time and determine if there is any pain in a particular area. Then, have the patient palpate beneath the patella for the patellar tendon, medially for medial collateral ligament, laterally for lateral collateral ligament, and inferiorly and medially for pes anserine bursa. Complete the palpation for both knees.

Sensation Testing
Ask the patient to lightly touch the upper thighs, lower thighs, inner shin, side of shin, top of foot, bottom of foot, on both sides

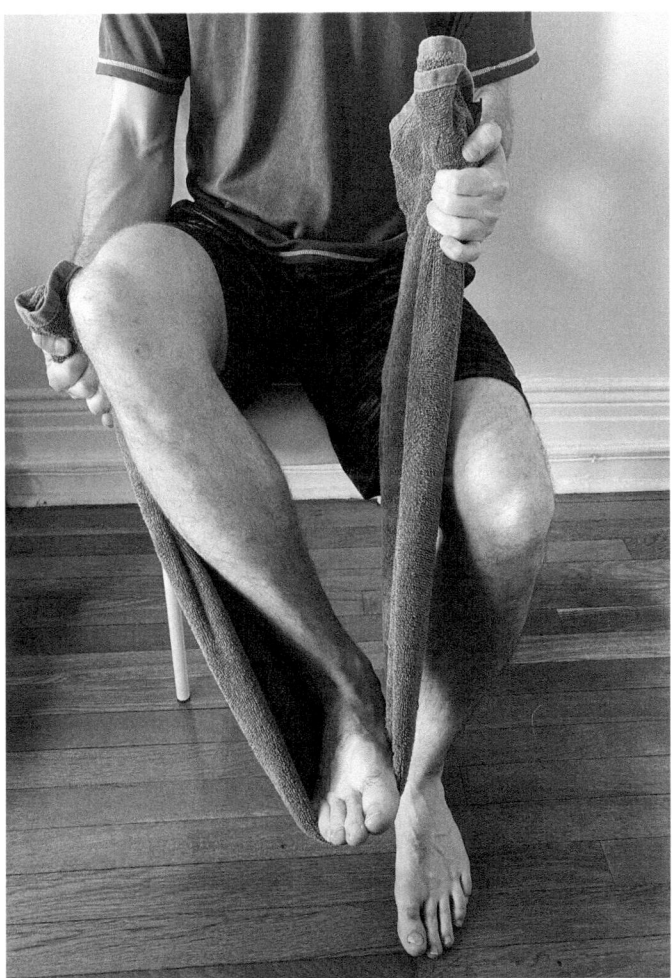

Fig. 11.3 Towel-assisted hip external rotation ROM testing

at the same time to compare light touch sensation. To test pin prick sensation, ask the patient to use a safety pin's sharp point in the same areas.

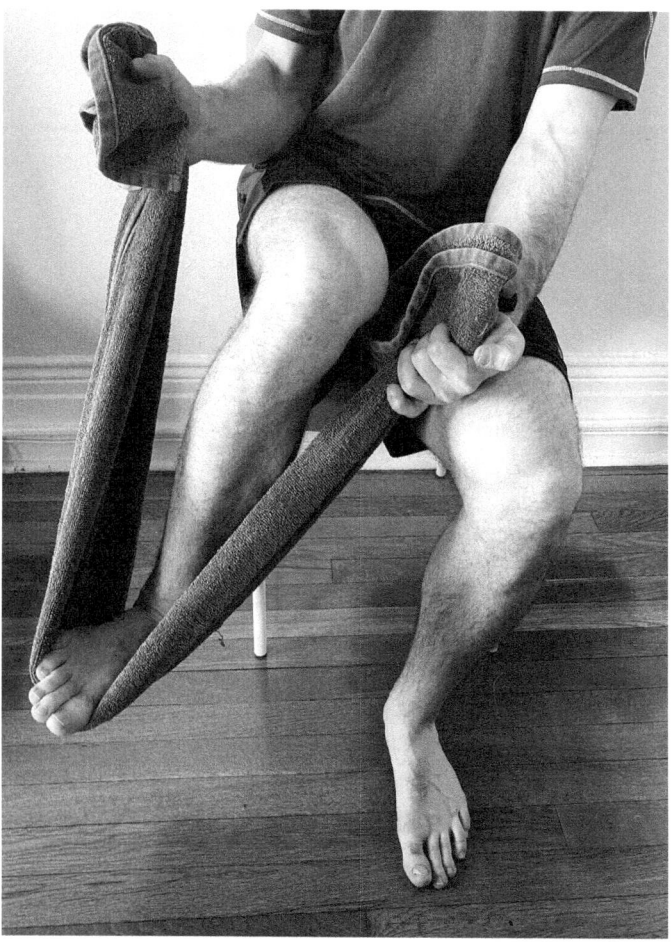

Fig. 11.4 Towel-assisted hip internal rotation ROM testing

Reflex Testing

To test patellar reflexes, have a small hand/face towel available. Have the patient feel for the bottom edge of the kneecap. Move slightly beneath the bony edge. Use the edge of a smartphone or television remote to lightly tap beneath the kneecap (Fig. 11.5). Use the small towel folded in half for a thin cushion as necessary. Test both sides.

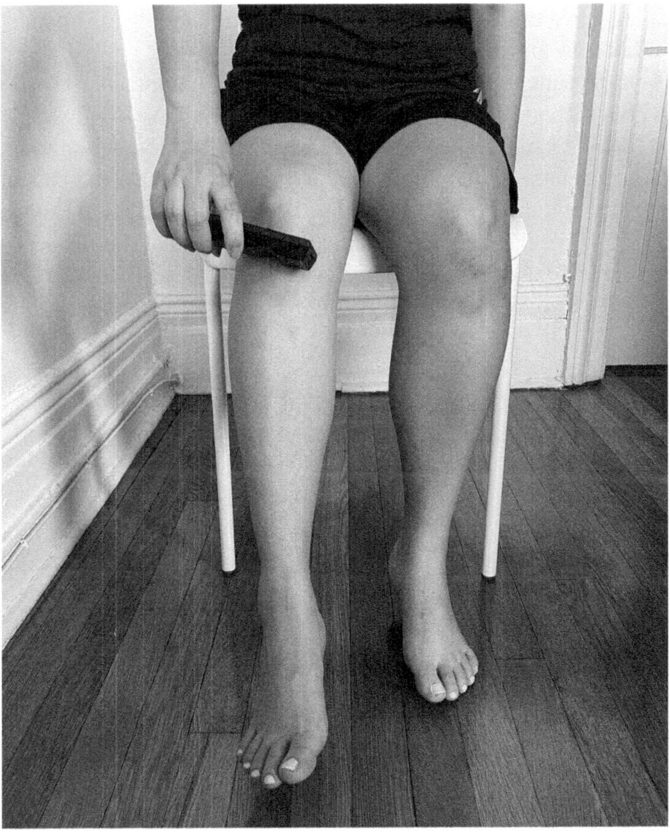

Fig. 11.5 Self patellar reflex testing with television remote

Strength Testing

To test for strength, have the patient perform a double-legged squat and a single-leg squat on each side. Check for the ability to return to standing and instability or inward rotation of the knee. The prior testing of active ROM with knee extension tested strength against gravity. Have the patient lift their ankles up and heel walk. Have the patient lift their big toe up one at a time. Then, have the patient stand on their tip toes and walk. If the patient is too unstable, ask them to pump their heels up and down at least five times. The previous would determine that the patient has at least antigravity strength.

If the patient has available resistance band equipment, strength with resistance can be tested. Have the patient hook a lightweight resistance band around a very sturdy table or closed in a door. Hooking the resistance band around the ankle, have the patient hip flex and then extend their knee on both sides (Figs. 11.6 and 11.7). While the patient is sitting down, change the position of the resistance band to the top of the foot and test dorsiflexion (Fig. 11.8).

Provocative Testing

Seated Provocative Testing [2]

For varus stress, have the patient use their top of the foot to hook around the other ankle and pull to the side (Fig. 11.9).

For valgus stress, have the patient use the bottom of their foot to push on the inner ankle of the other leg and push outward (Fig. 11.10).

Standing Provocative Testing

Duck Walk (Childress Test)
While fully squatting down, have the patient try and walk forwards, backwards, sideways. The patient can hold onto furniture if needed. Have the patient vocalize and localize any pain or clicking, or the inability to stay in the squat position.

Thessaly Test
While holding onto furniture, have the patient stand on one leg with foot flat on the ground and knee slightly bent. Ask them to rotate their body to twist around the knee. Have the patient vocalize and localize the pain. Repeat on the other side.

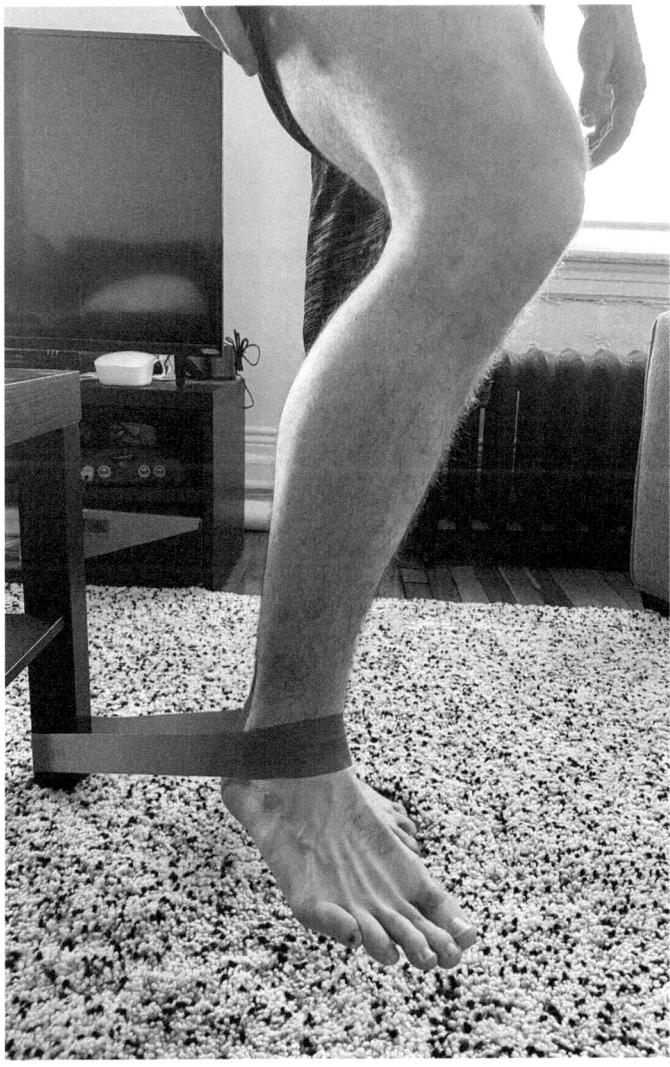

Fig. 11.6 Hip flexion strength testing against resistance

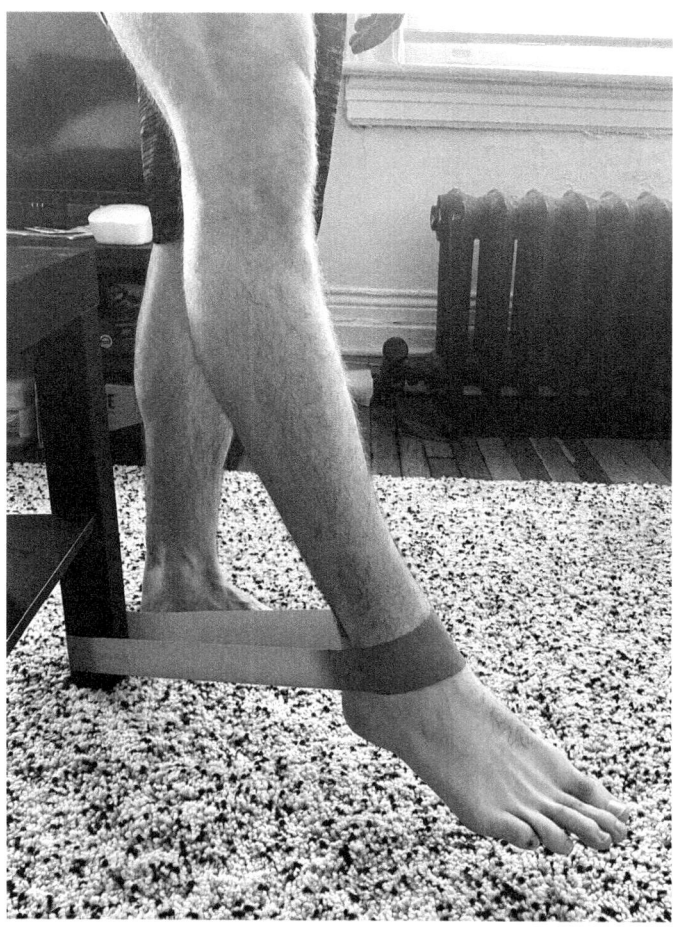

Fig. 11.7 Knee extension strength testing against resistance

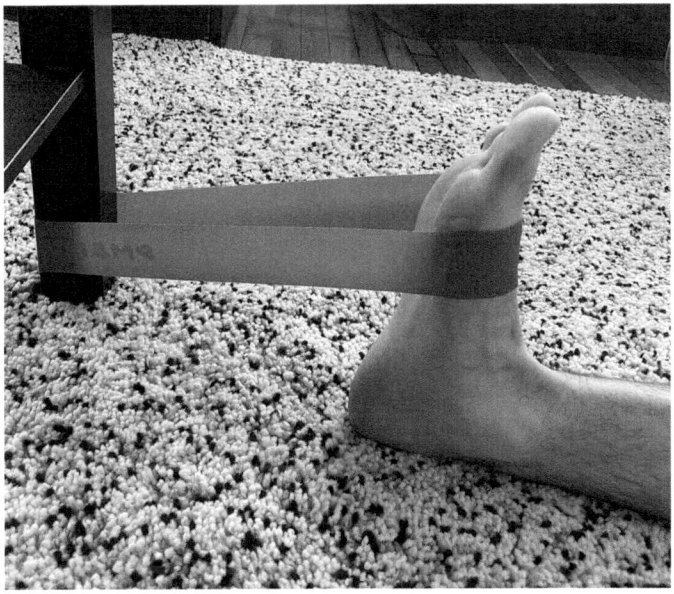

Fig. 11.8 Ankle dorsiflexion strength testing against resistance

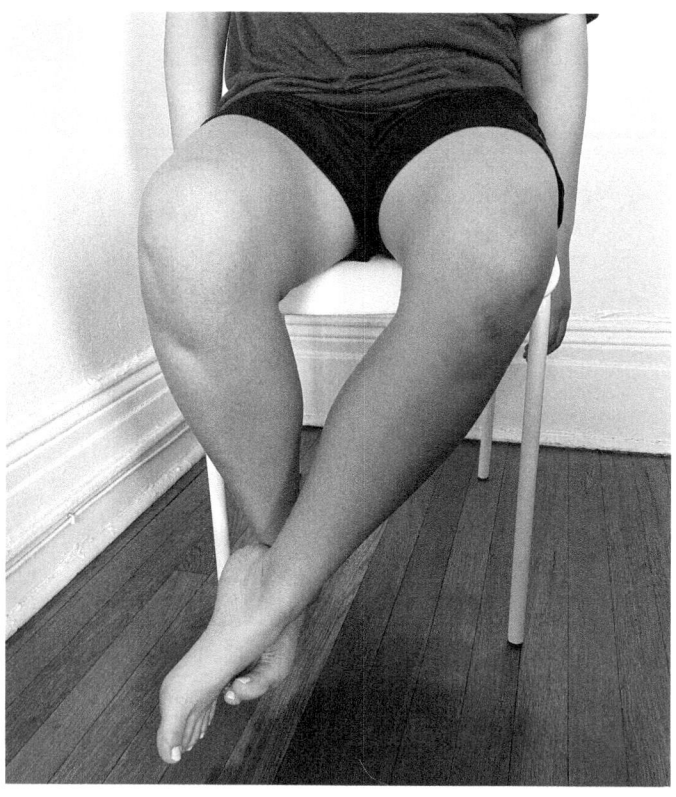

Fig. 11.9 Left knee self varus stress testing

11 The Telemedicine Knee Exam

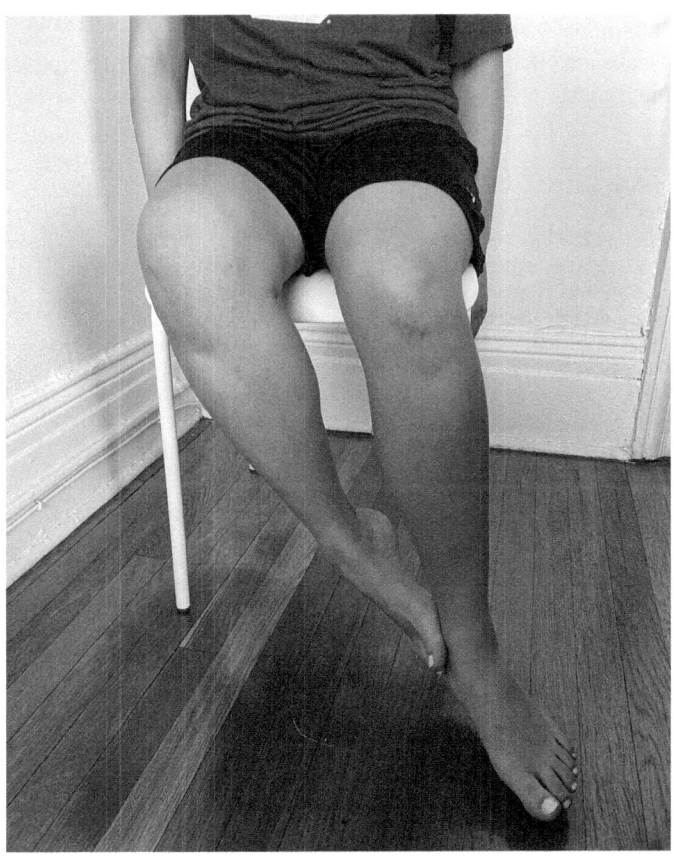

Fig. 11.10 Left knee self valgus stress testing

Differential Diagnoses

Please note that this is not a full nor extensive list of differential diagnoses.

Pediatric [3]	Adult [4]
• Bursitis • Cancer • Collateral ligament tear. Congenital malformations/deformity or mechanical, i.e., secondary to pes planus or genu valgum • Fracture • Hematologic disease • Idiopathic pain • Infectious arthritis, osteomyelitis • Legg–Calve–Perthes disease • Meniscus tear • Metabolic and endocrine disorders, i.e., rickets • Osgood–Schlatter disease • Patellar dislocation • Patellofemoral syndrome • Reactive/post-infectious arthritis • Rheumatologic disease, i.e., Kawasaki disease, lupus, juvenile idiopathic arthritis • Tendinopathy • Trauma	• Baker's cyst • Bursitis • Cancer • Collateral ligament tear • Congenital or acquired malformations/deformity or mechanical, i.e., secondary to pes planus or genu valgum • Crystal arthropathy • Fracture • Iliotibial band syndrome • Infectious arthritis, osteomyelitis • Meniscus tear • Osteoarthritis • Patellar dislocation • Patellofemoral syndrome • Pes anserine bursitis • Popliteal artery aneurysm • Radiating pain from the hip or back • Reactive arthritis • Rheumatologic disease, i.e., lupus, scleroderma Synovitis • Tendinopathy • Tendon tear • Trauma

Considerations for Specific Populations

For any clinical visit with a child, an adult should be present in the room to assist with the history and also examination. The adult will perform the examination as the assistant lined out above. To help with participation, toys or mobile device games can be given to the child while the adult is inspecting, palpating, testing motion. Try to avoid other distractions, such as siblings running throughout the room to ensure adequate participation of the child.

For older patients, it is important that they stay safe throughout the whole encounter. Using appropriate clinical judgment, certain testing, such as standing provocative tests, can be eliminated to reduce the risks for fall or further injury. It's also important to consider the patient population with visual or hearing impairments and how to accommodate them. Lastly, limitations due to body habitus should not be neglected.

Special Considerations

In addition to the importance of special populations, clinicians must also consider other factors that may affect a telemedicine evaluation. Pain is one of the common subjective indicators of the severity of an injury. Unlike during a traditional in-person physical examination, clinicians are unable to identify a patient's apprehension while knee ROM or provocative tests are performed either by the patient or assistant. Patients may be unwilling to have provocative tests performed by the assistant or there may be some hesitancy on behalf of the assistant in performing the task as well. Clinicians should provide reassurance and clear instructions need to be in place for all participants (patients and examiner).

Clinicians must also consider a patient's physical limitations that may affect their ability to perform certain parts of the physical examination. Some of these factors include: sensory deficits, spasticity, contractures, and/or heterotopic ossifications. Also keep in mind a patient's baseline level of function and medical conditions (spinal cord injury, peripheral neuropathy, peripheral arterial disease, limb amputation, etc.). Understanding these limitations will help guide clinicians on how to decipher new complaints from their baseline level of function. It is important to clarify with a patient the specific onset of a new complaint.

Management and Treatment

Although a telemedicine visit examination may not seem like an ideal encounter on which the management of a patient's chief complaint can be based, these visits are beneficial to clinicians and can be used as an initial screening encounter to determine proper follow-up care. Clinicians can determine the severity of an injury and whether it can be managed conservatively or surgically, and whether the joint needs further diagnostic testing or an in-person evaluation. Conservative management of an acute injury involves rest, ice, compression, and elevation. Pain management for less severe injuries could be by oral analgesics (NSAIDs), transdermal analgesic patches, or topical creams.

The Ottawa Knee rule, a simple ten question survey, along with physical examination can easily help determine if imaging of the knee is needed after acute trauma. This highly sensitive questionnaire can identify patients with fracture of the knee [5]. Although the questionnaire is designed for adults, it may also be applicable to children.

Clinicians can also decide on adjustments to weight bearing status based on their evaluation and make recommendations such as the use of crutches, changes to footwear, adaptations or precaution with walking up and down stairs. These patients should be offered a sooner follow-up or an in-person visit to decide the next step in management.

Clinicians can also make referrals for physical therapy sessions and provide timely follow-up to assess a patient's progress. For more emergent cases, clinicians can also determine which cases require an in-person visit or referral to an orthopedic surgeon for operative management.

Complications and Red Flags

There are several red flags to consider when evaluating patients for knee pain. Malignancies such as primary bone tumors (osteosarcoma, chondrosarcoma, and Ewing's sarcoma) can present as low grade pain and possible joint effusion accompanied by systemic symptoms such as fevers, chills, night sweats, and unintentional weight loss. Nocturnal bone pain is also an additional concerning complaint. Patients with these symptoms warrant an in-person evaluation, in-depth workup, and proper referral to an oncologist when there is a high level of suspicion.

Septic arthritis is another condition associated with joint effusion that is unrelated to activity, accompanied systemic signs (fever, chills, etc.). Unlike malignancies, patients with septic arthritis present with joint erythema and warmth. Diagnosis would involve immediate in-person evaluation, joint aspiration, fluid analysis, and antibiotics [4].

There are unique red flags to consider in the pediatric populations. Nocturnal joint and persistent bone pain are indicators of a malignancy. With malignant or infectious diseases children may present with complaints of malaise, reduced appetite, sweating, lethargy, and pallor in addition to the typical systemic signs [3].

Obvious changes that are a disruption of the normal structural anatomy warrant further evaluation. Signs of trauma such as hematoma or hemarthrosis may be indicators of injury to deeper tissues and structural components of the knee (bone, connective tissue, meniscus, fat pad, etc.). Referred pain may be an indicator of a hip pathology, while paresthesias may suggest a radiculopathy or peripheral nerve entrapment.

Follow-Up

As previously indicated, telemedicine visits can serve as a screening method to determine if a patient's chief complaint warrants an in-person visit, a closer follow-up, a referral to an orthopedic surgeon, or physical therapy. For minor musculoskeletal injuries that can be managed conservatively and do not require any imaging, patients can ideally be seen within 3 months, but this is left up to the clinician's discretion based on the injury. The decision as to whether the follow-up visit should be in-person or a telemedicine visit depends on factors such as logistics, concerns for progression of the injury, and the clinician's level of suspicion for differential diagnosis that may require a closer follow-up.

References

1. Malanga GA, Mautner K. Musculoskeletal physical examination. Amsterdam: Elsevier; 2017. p. 173–98.

2. Laskowski ER, Johnson SE, Shelerud RA, Lee JA, Rabatin AE, Driscoll SW, Moore BJ, Wainberg MC, Terzic CM. The telemedicine musculoskeletal examination. Mayo Clin Proc. 2020;95(8):1715–31. https://doi.org/10.1016/j.mayocp.2020.05.026.
3. Kimura Y, Southwood TR. Evaluation of the child with joint pain and/or swelling. Waltham: UpToDate; 2018. https://www.uptodate.com/contents/evaluation-of-the-child-with-joint-pain-and-or-swelling
4. Cover CJ, Shmerling RH. Approach to the adult with unspecified knee pain. Waltham: UpToDate; 2018. https://www.uptodate.com/contents/approach-to-the-adult-with-unspecified-knee-pain
5. Beutel BG, Trehan SK, Shalvoy RM, Mello MJ. The Ottawa knee rule: examining use in an academic emergency department. West J Emerg Med. 2012;13(4):366–72. https://doi.org/10.5811/westjem.2012.2.6892.

The Telemedicine Foot and Ankle Exam

12

Christopher Clifford, Liam J. Rawson, Lissa Hewan-Lowe, and Amie M. Kim

The foot and ankle exam provides clinically valuable information that can and should be preserved over a telehealth platform. The first critical skill is an understanding of the in-person exam, which can then be modified into a virtual version. The classic exam becomes that of a virtual interaction, and a provider's systematic approach supports successful patient participation while garnering necessary information. This chapter will overview the complete telemedicine foot and ankle history and physical, with a unique emphasis on the virtual environment.

C. Clifford (✉)
Department of Emergency Medicine, Mount Sinai Icahn School of Medicine, New York, NY, USA

L. J. Rawson
Department of Emergency Medicine, Mount Sinai Morningside / West, New York, NY, USA
e-mail: liam.rawson@mountsinai.org

L. Hewan-Lowe
Department of Physical Medicine Rehabilitation, Mount Sinai Icahn School of Medicine, New York, NY, USA

A. M. Kim
Department of Emergency Medicine, Department of Physical Medicine Rehabilitation, Icahn School of Medicine at Mount Sinai at Beth Israel, New York, NY, USA
e-mail: amie.kim@mountsinai.org

Chief Complaint and History of Present Illness

The common chief complaints for foot and ankle injury include: pain, swelling, deformity, stiffness, instability, or problem with gait [1]. A complete medical history is required. These questions include: occupation, athletic participation, inciting activity, and history of predisposing medical conditions that may manifest in the lower extremities including diabetes, neuropathy, peripheral vascular disease, inflammatory arthropathy, rheumatoid arthritis, vasculitis, or any prior or chronic injury.

Pain

Given the surface anatomy of the foot and ankle, identifying the location of pain is the first step. The patient can demonstrate the site of maximum pain. Define the pain as acute or chronic, elicit preceding events, characterize the pain (sharp, electric, dull, etc.), presence and degree of radiation (to the toes or up the leg), severity on a scale of 1–10, daytime variation of pain (first thing in the morning, after walking on it all day, in the middle of the night, etc.), and additional pain patterns such as predictable, reproducible, intermittent, or random. Next, ask the patient for aggravating and alleviating factors. Do they feel it more walking on a flat or uneven floor, ascending or descending stairs, worse with high heels or barefoot, relationship to weight bearing, better with rest, ice, or any additional remedies the patient has tried. Lastly, it is important to ask the patient what they believe is causing his pain [2].

Swelling

The patient can demonstrate the area of greatest swelling. Determine whether the swelling is painful or painless. Is it the result of an acute versus overuse injury. Identify the timeline when the swelling first began and its progression. Characterize associated skin changes, whether the swelling is firm or fluctuant, and if there has been recent change in footwear or activity. Confirm that the swelling is unilateral and not generalized or bilateral. A bilateral swelling of the feet and ankles often signifies cardiac, renal, or hepatic pathology.

As always, red flag symptoms must be eliminated. These include infection, neoplastic/spinal processes, and vascular compromise. Questions to ask the patient include: night sweats, fever, pain out of proportion to exam, decreased range of motion, weight loss, numbness, weakness, dusky foot, black discoloration at the tips of the toes.

The Virtual Exam of the Foot and Ankle

We suggest a stepwise approach to completing the physical exam with the structure as follows: initial setup, inspection, palpation, range of motion, neurologic and vascular exam, strength testing, reflex testing, special testing.

Initial Setup

The patient adjusts the camera so that the foot and ankle is fully visualized. This can be challenging when it comes to the lower half of the body. Placing the camera on the floor or on a small stool or chair provides an eye level view. If a family member or friend is available, ask them to assist by filming the patient during the physical exam. Confirm adequate space for the patient to walk at least three steps forward and backwards. Ensure adequate lighting in the room and that shadows are not causing interference. Encourage the patient to introduce additional light sources [3].

The patient should wear loose fitting shorts that allows complete exposure of both legs from above the knees to the bottom of the feet in both sitting and standing positions. Socks and shoes should be removed for the entirety of the exam. Confirm that the patient is comfortable with the level of exposure and adjust accordingly.

Inspection

Initial observation begins with bilateral exposure and gross comparison from the anterior, posterior, and lateral positions (see anterior, posterior, lateral right, and lateral left views below). If the patient can negotiate standing, the patient can place the camera on the ground or a small stool and turn in a circle. If the patient cannot stand, the patient can sit in a chair and place both feet flat on the ground. The patient spins the camera around the feet and ankles to view all sides. Lastly, if possible, the patient can lay supine with the camera oriented to the bottom of the feet in an axial projection (Fig. 12.1).

Assess for structural symmetry and any gross deformities of bilateral feet and ankles. Look for skin changes such as erythema and ecchymosis. Identify joint effusions with attention to the ankle. Look for muscle atrophy throughout, in particular the calf muscles. Note deviations from neutral anatomy including equinus contracture, and in bony alignment including varus or valgus hindfoot, cavus or planus midfoot, forefoot adduction or abduction, hallux varus or valgus, and claw or mallet deformities of the lesser toes.

Palpation

Instruct the seated patient to palpate his ankle and foot to identify areas of pain. Start on a single calf moving down the leg towards the ankle using one or both hands (see calf palpation below). Repeat at the alternate calf to compare sides. Repeat circumferentially at each ankle. Palpate each foot on both the top and bottom. Lastly, palpate each individual toe. Key bony, ligamentous, and tendinous landmarks that should be individually palpated include: the fibula, anterior and posterior talofibular ligaments, deltoid ligament, calcaneofibular ligament, talar neck, lateral malleolus, medial malleolus, peroneal tendons, Achilles tendon, anterior ankle joint line, calcaneus, calcaneal tubercle, mid-foot, and fifth metatarsal. The anterior projection is best to view self-palpation of the medial malleolus and navicular bones. The lateral projection is best to view self-palpation of the fifth metatarsal and the lateral malleolus. The posterior projection is best to view self-palpation of the Achilles tendon and the calcaneus (see navicular, medial malleolus, lateral malleolus, calcaneal, and Achilles tendon palpation below) (Fig. 12.2).

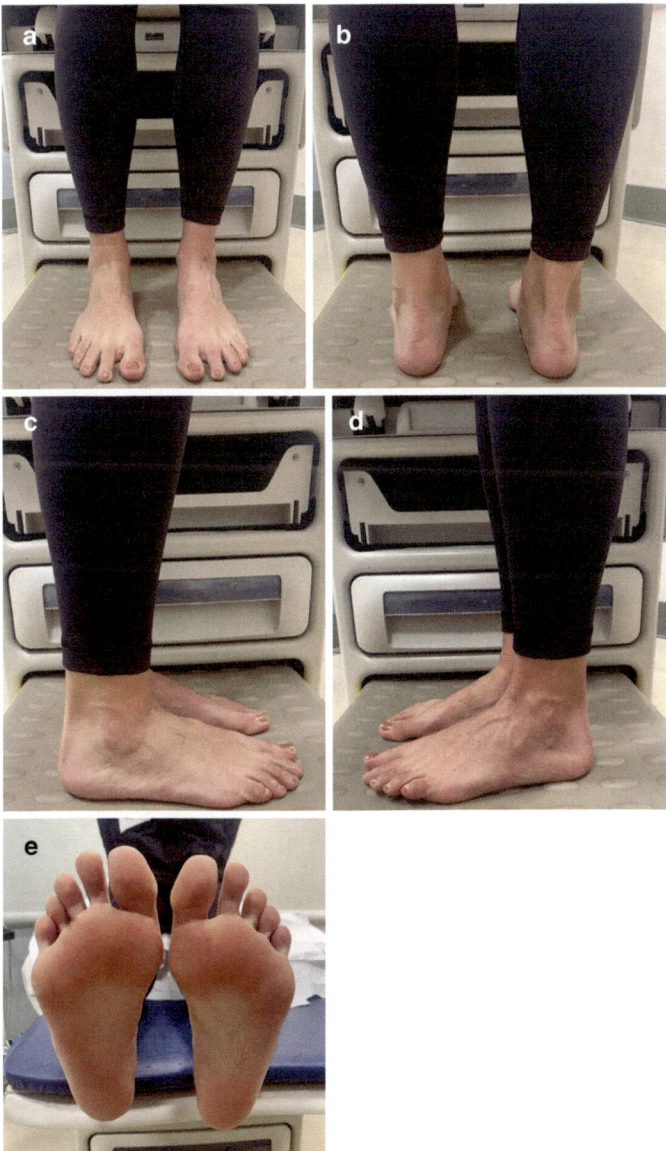

Fig. 12.1 (**a**) Anterior view. (**b**) Posterior view. (**c**) Lateral right view. (**d**) Lateral left view. (**e**) Axial view

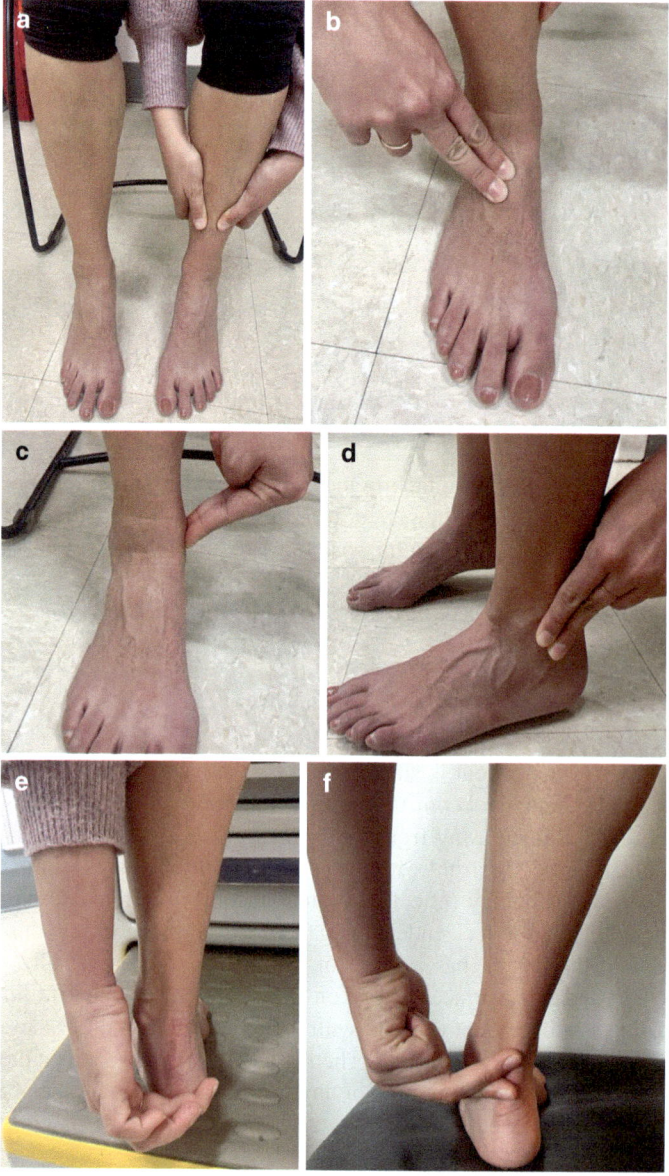

Fig. 12.2 (**a**) Calf palpation. (**b**) Navicular palpation. (**c**) Medial malleolus palpation. (**d**) Lateral malleolus palpation. (**e**) Calcaneal palpation. (**f**) Achilles tendon palpation

Range of Motion

Active range of motion (ROM) can be assessed in both standing and seated positions but seated may be preferred to prevent loss of balance. A web or app-based goniometer may be used by the patient to measure precise degrees of motion. Moderate to excellent correlation in ankle ROM has been demonstrated between smartphone-based virtual goniometry and in-person goniometry [4].

Instruct the patient to plantarflex and dorsiflex the ankle. Normal ROM is 50° and 20°, respectively. Evaluate subtalar ROM with the patient in a seated crossed position with the foot over the knee. With one hand, stabilize the ankle and with the other hand, apply gentle inversion and eversion stresses to lateral and medial foot. Normal ROM is 35° and 25°, respectively (see ankle inversion and eversion below). Lastly, have the patient flex and extend the toes. A common and quick alternative to evaluate gross ROM is to ask the patient to draw an air circle with their toes, thereby ranging the ankle in all directions in a single movement (Fig. 12.3).

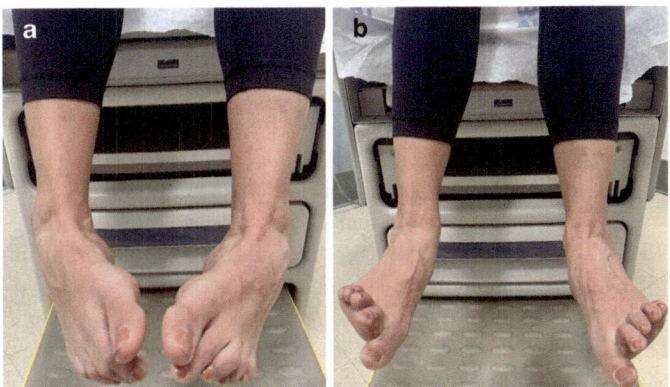

Fig. 12.3 (**a**) Ankle inversion. (**b**) Ankle eversion

Neurologic and Vascular Examination

The patient may be able to identify their dorsalis pedis pulse with instruction. It is commonly palpable at the dorsum of the foot in the first intermetatarsal space immediately lateral to the extensor hallucis longus. If the patient has their finger in the correct location but does not feel the pulse, instruct them to apply varying degrees of pressure until a pulse is felt. The patient can be coached to perform capillary refill testing. Ask them to pinch their toe and demonstrate the technique on the fingers of your own hand. The provider views and counts capillary refill time. If the patient appreciates discoloration in their foot, they should raise the foot above the level of the heart to see if discoloration subsequently resolves. If it does not, infection or arterial compromise may be suspected.

Sensation can be assessed by asking the patient to touch both feet simultaneously and assess if it feels the same on both sides. Finger sensation is a confounder so utilizing an object (e.g., a pencil or brush for light touch and a safety pin for pin prick) may be beneficial.

Strength Testing

Reliable strength assessment is challenging for the patient to self-perform in the virtual musculoskeletal exam of the foot and ankle, but range of resistance can be standardized to elicit strength objectivity. Begin by observing the patient's gait through several steps. Next, observe the patient's gait while walking on tiptoes. Toe walk indicates at least a 4/5 strength in ankle plantarflexion [5]. Observe patient's gait with a single foot on tiptoe (see single foot tiptoe below). Single foot toe hop indicates a 5/5 strength in ankle plantarflexion. Dorsiflexion may be tested with the patient seated, and ankle dorsiflexed against a vertical surface (see vertical surface dorsiflexed below). This indicates at least a 3/5 strength for ankle dorsiflexion. Note that single leg maneuvers limit the evaluation of asymmetries. The clinician can coach a family

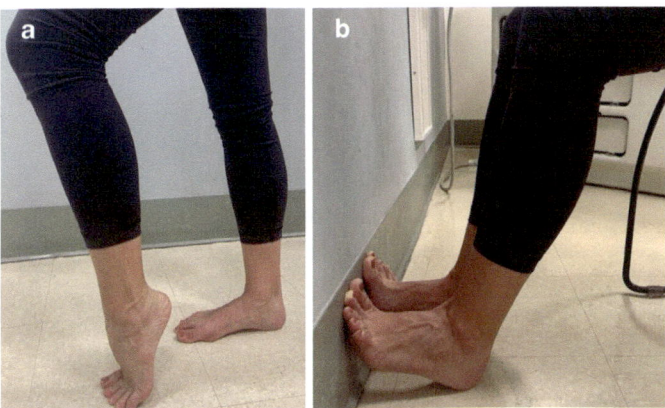

Fig. 12.4 (a) Single foot tiptoe. (b) Vertical surface dorsiflexed

member or friend to simultaneously assess both sides and report on symmetry observed (Fig. 12.4).

Inversion and eversion resistance testing can be evaluated against a vertical surface like a wall or table leg. Ankle eversion is tested by planting lateral aspect of the patient's forefoot against the stationary surface, while exerting a rotational push into the surface. Ankle inversion is tested by planting the medial aspect of the patient's big toe against the stationary surface, while exerting a rotational push into the surface [3], (see inversion and eversion telemedicine + anatomic maneuver below) (Fig. 12.5).

Reflex Testing

Reflex testing is challenging for the patient to self-perform as patients often increase the muscle tone of the structure of interest in anticipation of the object striking their body. Engaging a family member or friend in this scenario can be helpful. To test the Achilles tendon reflex, instruct the assistant to elevate the patient's foot by cupping his hand at the patient's heel. Using a firm edge (e.g., smartphone, rubber spatula, etc.) to gently strike the Achilles tendon. The exam is per-

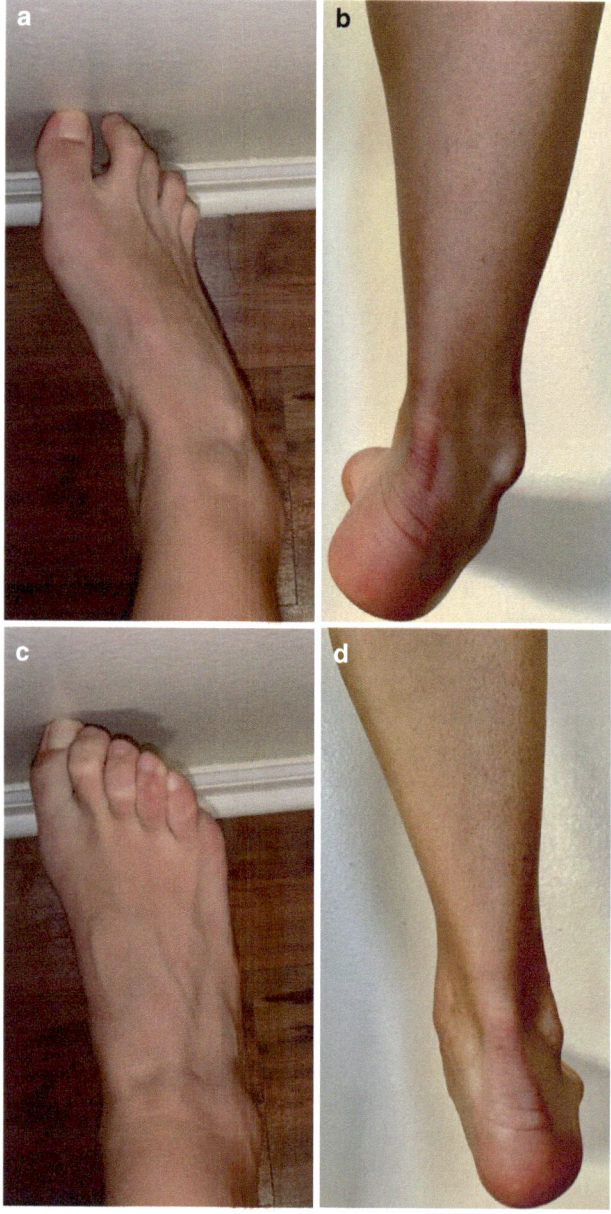

Fig. 12.5 Inversion: (**a**) Telemedicine maneuver. (**b**) Anatomic maneuver. Eversion: (**c**) Telemedicine maneuver. (**d**) Anatomic maneuver

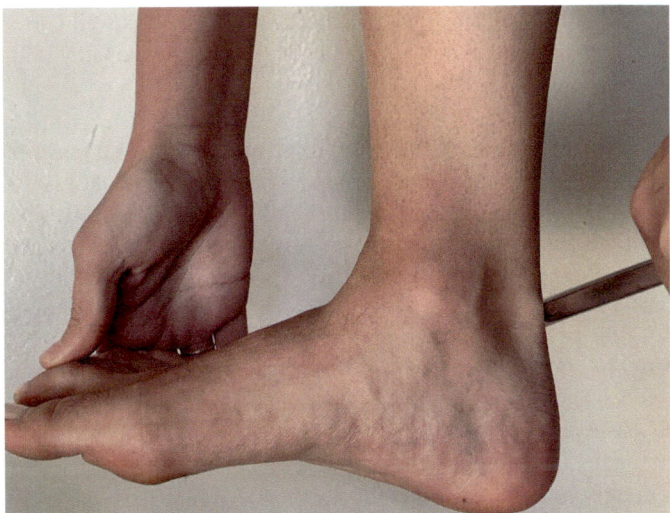

Fig. 12.6 Achilles tendon reflex

formed bilaterally, and the clinician observes for the appropriate reflex (see Achilles tendon reflex below) (Fig. 12.6).

Special Tests

This section includes tests that can be performed in the seated position versus standing or walking. The camera angle will need to change significantly with each position change.

Seated Special Tests

Thompson Test

Evaluates Achilles Tendon Rupture

Patient kneels backwards on a chair with the knee in 90° flexion. Patient reaches back and locates their calf with the ipsilateral hand. Patient is instructed to squeeze until they see or feel their ankle begin to plantarflex. Set up the camera lateral to the patient

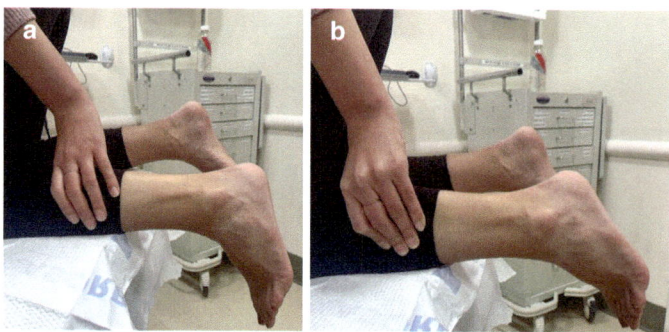

Fig. 12.7 (**a**) Thompson test begin. (**b**) Thompson test end

to observe the degree of plantar flexion. Remind the patient to maintain postural balance during this maneuver [3], (see Thompson test begin and end below) (Fig. 12.7).

Anterior Drawer Test

Evaluates Anterior Talofibular Ligament Laxity

Patient is in a seated crossed position with the foot over the knee. Patient takes one hand to the anterior, distal leg while the second-hand cups the heel and brings the ankle into passive plantarflexion. Translate the heel anteriorly to assess for pain and laxity (see anterior drawer test below) (Fig. 12.8).

Talar Tilt

Evaluates Talar Instability

Patient is in a seated crossed position with the foot over the knee. Patient takes one hand to the medial, distal leg while the second-hand cups the hindfoot and brings the ankle into passive 15° of

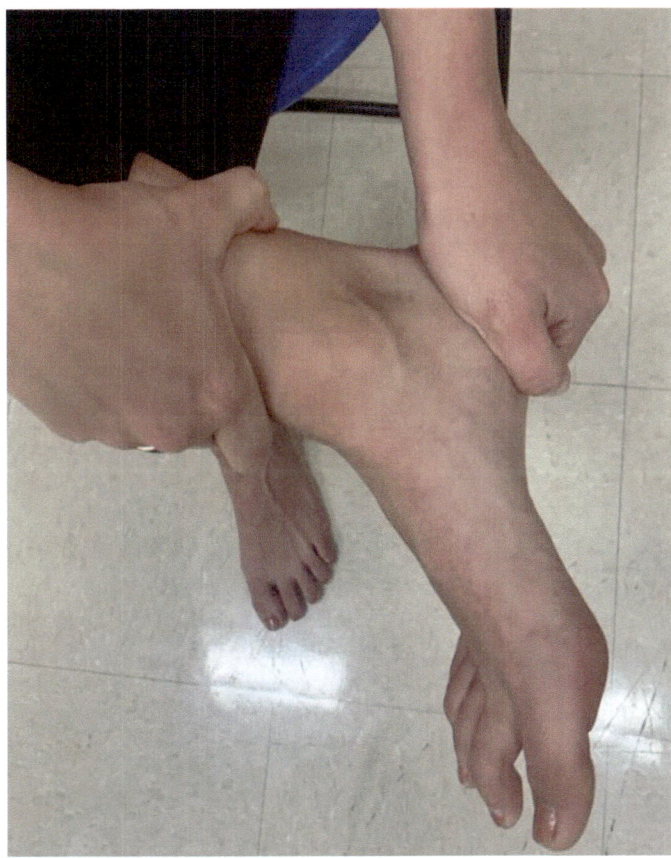

Fig. 12.8 Anterior drawer test

plantarflexion, then applies an inversion force. Assess for pain and laxity (see talar tilt test begin and end below) (Fig. 12.9).

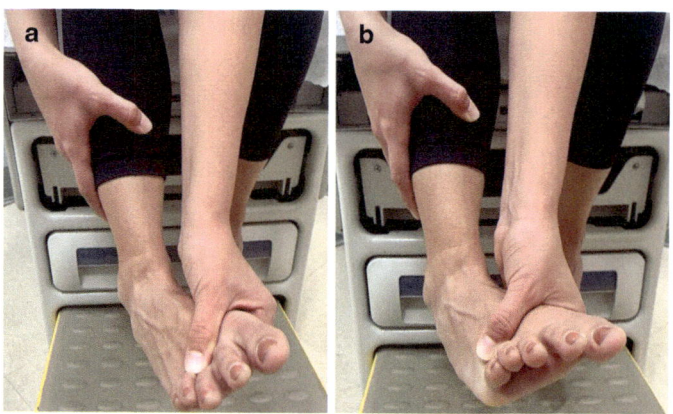

Fig. 12.9 (**a**) Talar tilt begin. (**b**) Talar tilt end

Metatarsal Squeeze

Evaluates Morton's or Interdigital Neuroma

Patient is in a seated crossed position with the foot over the knee. Patient places one hand just proximal to the toes and squeezes the forefoot from both sides. Patient's second-hand palpates between the third and fourth metatarsals assessing for pain or clicking (see metatarsal squeeze below) (Fig. 12.10).

Kleiger's Test

Evaluates for Medial Ankle Sprain

Patient is in a seated position with the foot and ankle hanging freely. Patient places one hand on the leg just proximal to the ankle to provide stability. Patient's second-hand grasps the midfoot keeping the ankle in a neutral position and then externally rotates the foot. The test is positive if pain is felt at the interosseous membrane or medial ankle (see Kleiger's test below) (Fig. 12.11).

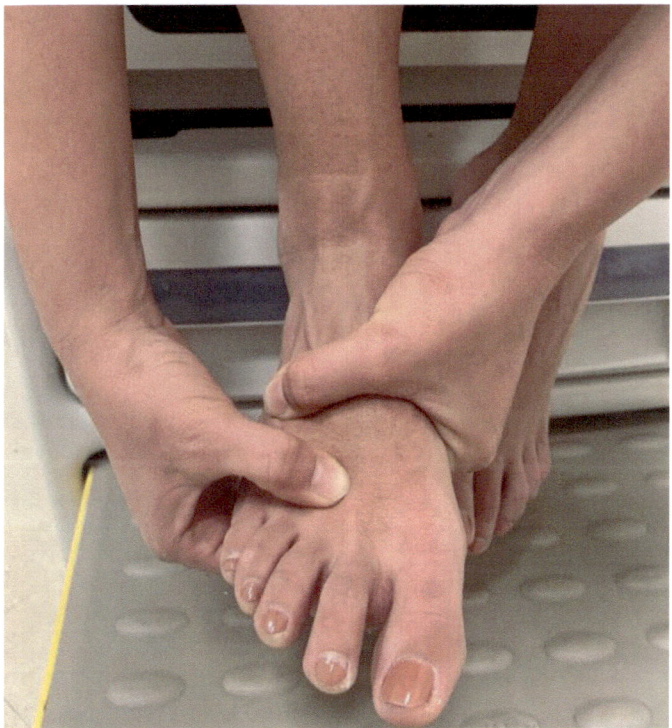

Fig. 12.10 Metatarsal squeeze

Standing or Walking Special Tests

Encourage the patient to perform these exam maneuvers next to a wall to maintain postural balance.

Coleman Block Test

Evaluates hindfoot flexibility and determines forefoot versus hindfoot-driven cavovarus foot.

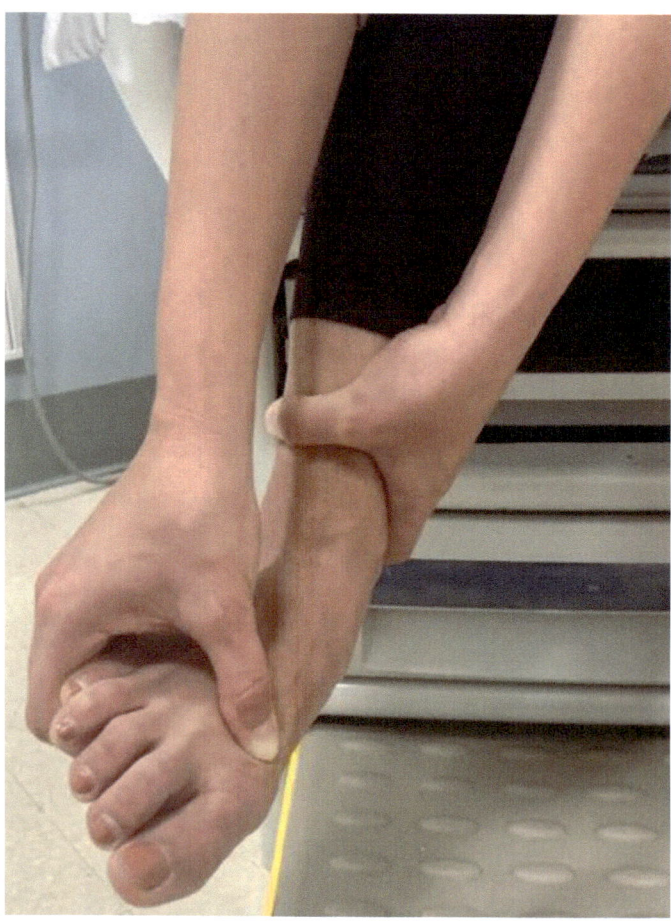

Fig. 12.11 Kleiger's test

Place the camera on the floor or a small stool so that the feet are in coronal view. Place a stack of magazines or a small book under the lateral border of the foot. As the patient weight bears into standing position, observe if the first metatarsal drops below the level of the item that is under the lateral foot. A drop indicates hindfoot flexibility and a forefoot-driven varus. If the first metatarsal does not drop below the level of the item, then this indicates

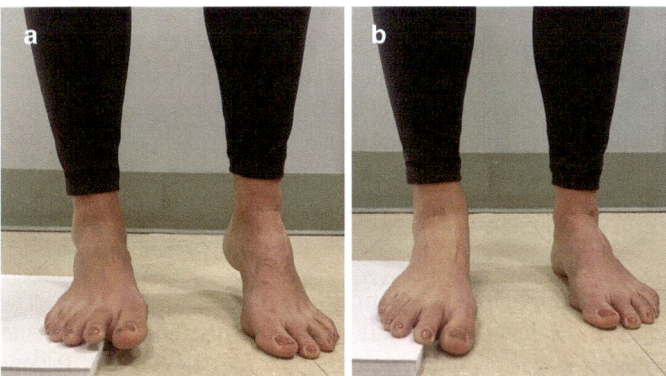

Fig. 12.12 (**a**) Coleman block test without drop. (**b**) Coleman block test with drop

hindfoot rigidity and hindfoot-driven varus [2], (see Coleman block test with and without drop below) (Fig. 12.12).

Gait Assessment

Place the camera on a small stool or on the floor to view the patient's lower extremities from hips to barefeet. Ensure the patient has adequate space. Observe their gait in walking three steps towards and away from the camera. Assess the hips for a Trendelenburg sign (unilateral hip drop), hip abduction or high angle footstep to compensate for a potential foot drop, and if the patient favors one foot over the other in antalgia. A side angle view with the camera is rarely helpful.

Tiptoe Walk

Evaluates plantarflexion strength, midfoot function, and S1–2 nerve function.

Place the camera on a small stool or on the floor to view the patient's lower extremities from upper legs to barefeet. Patient stands on tiptoes and toe walks away from the camera, turns, and then returns towards camera view. Assess antalgic toe walk gait or any localized pain. Pain in the posterior medial heel may indicate posterior tibialis tendinitis. Pain in the midfoot may indicate stress fracture or Lisfranc complex injury.

Heel Walk

Evaluates L4–5 Nerve Function

Place the camera on a small stool or on the floor to view the patient's lower extremities from upper legs to barefeet. Patient stands on hind feet and heel walks away from the camera, turns, and then returns towards camera view. Assess antalgic heel walk gait or any localized pain. Pain in the anterior ankle may indicate anterior tibialis tendinitis. Pain at the plantar aspect may indicate plantar fasciitis.

Hop Test

Evaluates Power and Strength Usually Before Return to Sports Post-injury

Place the camera on a small stool or on the floor to view the patient's lower extremities from upper legs to barefeet. Patient stands on one foot while using a wall for balance and hops vertically off one foot. Assess both sides and look for asymmetry in strength or balance. The hop test can be modified as needed per athletic ability. Evaluating distance traveled in a single hop or speed at which a course can be completed while hopping may allow evaluation virtually.

Special Populations

Postoperative patients are at risk for complications, and on-site evaluations are encouraged. However, a virtual exam can provide valuable information while supporting patient safety and comfort during the recovery period. Visualization and self-palpation of the surgical site should be completed to evaluate wound dehiscence, drainage, erythema, swelling, warmth, or tenderness. A neurovascular exam can be performed as above. Range of motion, strength testing, gait assessment, and other special exams may be severely limited while causing injury to a healing site [5].

Differential Diagnosis

The initial differential diagnosis is driven by a detailed history and location of pain (Tables 12.1 and 12.2).

Management and Treatment

Management of foot and ankle injuries are largely driven by diagnosis and severity of injury, and there may be utility in obtaining radiology and initiating protective immobilization. The time

Table 12.1 List of common ankle injuries as organized by the presence or absence of injury on history and location of pain on exam

Medial ankle pain	Anterior ankle pain
Injury:	Injury:
1. Deltoid ligament injury	1. Articular surface injury
2. Medial malleolus stress fracture	2. Tibialis anterior tendon rupture
No injury:	No injury:
1. Tibialis posterior tendonitis	1. Tibialis anterior tendinopathy
2. Tarsal tunnel syndrome	2. Anterior ankle impingement
Lateral ankle pain	Posterior ankle pain
Injury:	Injury:
1. Lateral ligament sprain	1. Achilles tendon partial/full rupture
2. Distal fibula or cuboid stress fracture	2. Fracture of talar process
3. Lateral talar process fracture	No injury:
4. Inferior tibiofibular joint injury	1. Achilles tendinitis
No injury:	2. Flexor hallucis tendonitis
1. Peroneal tendonitis	
2. Peroneal tendon subluxation	

Table 12.2 List of common foot injuries as organized by location of pain on exam

Heel pain	Midfoot pain
1. Plantar fasciitis 2. Heel spurs 3. Haglund deformity 4. Achilles tendinopathy 5. Calcaneal stress fracture	1. Tarsal tunnel syndrome 2. Excessive pronation 3. Navicular stress fracture 4. Lisfranc injuries
Arch pain	Forefoot pain
1. Flat foot 2. High arches	1. Morton's neuroma 2. Hallux valgus/rigidus 3. Metatarsal stress fracture 4. Metatarsalgia 5. Toe deformities

course in obtaining radiographic information can be driven by your practice infrastructure and clinical urgency. Consider empiric immobilization or supportive orthosis until these data result, while protecting further injury, managing symptoms, and promoting functionality. An illustrative example is included below in the management of low ankle sprain.

If an uncomplicated low ankle sprain is suspected, the PRICE protocol (protected weight bearing, rest, ice, compression, and elevation) may be initiated. 72-hours rest post-injury is recommended, with gradual reintegration of activity as tolerated by symptoms. Patients with access to crutches may be permitted to use these initially for comfort and correct fit and crutch training can be performed virtually. However, patients with minor sprains should be encouraged to resume activities with early protected weight bearing (CAM boot, air cast, ankle lace up, or elastic bandage) as this has been shown to improve recovery time and functional activity [6]. During the initial 48 h post-injury, patients should frequently elevate the affected extremity above heart level and apply compressive elastic bandage to reduce swelling. Pain control can be achieved with nonsteroidal anti-inflammatory drugs or acetaminophen if not contraindicated. Ice may also be applied for swelling reduction and symptomatic relief [6]. Early rehabilitation such as air drawing the alphabet with the toes and towel pick-ups is suggested to improve ankle joint range of

Table 12.3 List of common red flag signs and symptoms

Signs of severe or rapidly spreading infection
Pain out of proportion to exam
Night sweats or fever
Open wound with exposed tendon/ligaments/bone
Signs of malignancy such as weight loss and incontinence
Signs of necrosis
Severe discoloration (dusky, black)
Loss of sensation
Paresis or paralysis
Gross deformity or malalignment
Inability to bear weight

motion, strength and function and to reduce recurrent instability [6].

Red Flags

With red flag symptoms or signs, the patient and/or caregiver should be referred immediately to the emergency department for evaluation and treatment. Coordination of emergency services can include arranging transportation, communicating with the receiving emergency department providers, or sending additional documentation. Below is a list of the most common red flags that must be identified and addressed immediately (Table 12.3).

Complications

Below is a list of common complications associated with foot and ankle injuries that require a high index of suspicion during evaluation.

Infection

Necrotizing fasciitis and septic joint must be considered. Things to clue you off for necrotizing fasciitis include immunocompromised host, rapid spread of infection, and pain out of proportion to exam. A patient with septic joint may report night sweats, joint effusion, and exquisite pain with passive ROM.

Neoplasm

A neoplastic process in the spine should be considered, especially in the elderly. Patients can present with foot and ankle chief complaints later identified as a secondary process to compressive mass lesions of the spinal nerves. Red flags that should be considered include a history of cancer (particularly prostate), weight loss, numbness, weakness, and change in gait, bladder or bowel function.

Vascular Compromise

Since the foot is the most distal structure of the body, often patients with significant arterial pathology will present with foot or ankle complaints as sentinel signs. Two emergent signs are the dusky discoloration of the foot or a black discoloration at the tips of the toes. However, loss of sensation and paralysis can be late signs of vascular compromise.

Fracture and Dislocation

There are several worrisome fractures and dislocations that if missed can result in significant morbidity. Most patients with occult fractures will report inciting trauma, significant subsequent pain, gross deformity, inability to bear weight, swelling, or bruising. Joint dislocations of the foot and ankle are typically high energy injuries, but a single toe phalanx dislocation may be subtle. A Lisfranc fracture may present with bruising to the arch and swelling of the mid foot. Most fractures and dislocations require emergent closed reduction and immobilization.

Follow-Up

Telemedicine for the foot and ankle can be of high utility to clinicians while comfortable for patients after the initial on-site evaluation. Well-visits or post-procedural patients may present a particularly high yield opportunity to review imaging results and perform interval reassessment.

References

1. Reider B. The orthopaedic physical examination. 2nd ed. Amsterdam: Elsevier Saunders; 2005. p. 383.
2. Alazzawi S, Sukeik M, King D, Vemulapalli K. Foot and ankle history and clinical examination: a guide to everyday practice. World J Orthop. 2017;8(1):21–9. https://doi.org/10.5312/wjo.v8.i1.21.
3. Laskowski ER, et al. The telemedicine musculoskeletal examination. Mayo Clin Proc. 2020;95(8):1715–31. https://doi.org/10.1016/j.mayocp.2020.05.026.
4. Wang KY, Hussaini SH, Teasdall RD, Gwam CU, Scott AT. Smartphone applications for assessing ankle range of motion in clinical practice. Foot Ankle Orthop. 2019;4(3):2473011419874779.
5. Eble SK, Hansen OB, Ellis SJ, Drakos MC. The virtual foot and ankle physical examination. Foot Ankle Int. 2020;41(8):1017–26. https://doi.org/10.1177/1071100720941020.
6. Melanson SW, Shuman VL. Acute ankle sprain. Treasure Island (FL): StatPearls Publishing; 2020.

Telemedicine Evaluation and Management of Respiratory Muscle Dysfunction

Michael Chiou, John R. Bach, and Charles Kent

There are 45 respiratory muscles and their dysfunction can often be adequately assessed and managed by a telemedicine visit. This chapter serves to inform the reader about telemedicine assessment and management of adults with respiratory muscle dysfunction causing ventilatory pump failure (VPF). While an in-person assessment optimizes the clinician's opportunity to perform a comprehensive examination and provide patient education, life-preserving interventions *can* be prescribed during a telemedicine visit. In this chapter, we will focus on the respiratory muscles—the diaphragm and other muscles of respiration.

The standard of care is to treat airway secretion accumulation and high CO_2 with noninvasive ventilatory support (NVS) and mechanical insufflation–exsufflation (MIE). Previously, patients

---

M. Chiou (✉) · C. Kent
Department of Rehabilitation and Human Performance, Icahn School of Medicine at Mount Sinai, New York, NY, USA

J. R. Bach
Department of Physical Medicine and Rehabilitation, Rutgers New Jersey Medical School, Newark, NJ, USA
e-mail: bachjr@njms.rutgers.edu

with weak respiratory muscles were instead provided supplemental O_2 to treat them for sleep disordered breathing. However, we now know that O_2 and/or sedative medications can increase blood CO_2 levels by over 150 mmHg, which can lead to hypercapnic acute ventilatory failure/acute respiratory failure (ARF). When chronic ventilatory insufficiency becomes acute ventilatory failure, the patient is intubated, that is, an endotracheal tube is passed through the nose or mouth and into the windpipe (trachea) for invasive ventilatory support and airway suctioning. While intubated, once the patient fails spontaneous breathing trials and ventilator weaning parameters, without the consent of the patient who is often medicated to remain unconscious, the family is often urged to consent to having a tracheostomy tube surgically inserted through the neck and into the trachea. The same ventilators and ventilator settings that are used for invasive mechanical ventilation could have been used for NVS delivery for noninvasive support, but clinicians do not use these ventilatory support settings via noninvasive tubes for NVS, which is why the patients are often unnecessarily intubated. Minimum span bi-level positive airway pressure (PAP) often does not prevent acute ventilatory failure, but NVS does. Patients can be managed by NVS and MIE rather than have to resort to tracheotomies if intubated and ventilator "unweanable."

Most patients with impairment of pulmonary function can be differentiated into (1) those who have primarily *oxygenation impairment* with hypoxemia resulting from intrapulmonary shunting due to intrinsic lung/airway disease and for which hypercapnia is an end-stage event due to dead space ventilation or (2) those with lung *ventilation impairment* on the basis of central hypoventilation from central respiratory controller hypoactivity, excessive work of breathing, or respiratory muscle dysfunction for whom hypoventilation causes hypoxia and hypercapnia. The distinction between respiratory and ventilatory impairment is important. Many patients in the former category have been described to benefit from "noninvasive ventilation" or "NIV" that has come to be synonymous with continuous positive airway pressure (CPAP) that does not directly assist weak respiratory muscles and low span (pressure support, drive pressure) bi-level PAP that is suboptimal and ultimately ineffective to prevent acute on chronic ventilatory/respiratory failure for patients with primarily ventilatory impairment and VPF since the minimal ventilatory assistance of NIV neither adequately rests respiratory muscles nor provides ventilatory support. Instead, patients with advanced VPF can benefit from the use of both inspiratory and expiratory muscle aids at NVS settings and MIE in the form of a CoughAssist™ (Respironics Inc., Murrysville, PA) to expel airway secretions when cough peak flows (CPF) are suboptimal. Thus, positive pressures applied to the airways during inspiration assist or support the inspiratory muscles just as negative pressure to the airways during expiration assists or supports the expiratory muscles to increase cough flows. Physical medicine interventions also include the application of pressures to the body to increase both inspiratory and expiratory muscle function (e.g., body ventilators).

Typical examples of ventilatory insufficiency include that of mildly hypercapnic patients with myopathic or lower motor neuron disorders who may have normal O_2 saturation when awake but are hypercapnic with O_2 desaturations during sleep unless using sleep NVS. Patients who become symptomatic from ventilatory insufficiency most often have daytime hypercapnia and dips in O_2 saturation below 95%, but their blood pH may remain normal due to compensatory metabolic alkalosis. Symptomatic hypercapnic patients benefit from extending the use of sleep NVS into daytime hours for at least part of the day. Severe ventilatory muscle weakness and need for NVS (where withdrawal from it results in immediate dyspnea and blood gas derangement) denotes ventilatory muscle failure which, if not treated by NVS and MIE, results in the extreme hypercapnia and decreased blood pH of acute ventilatory failure.

Ventilatory muscle failure is defined by the inability of the inspiratory and expiratory muscles to sustain one's respiration without resort to both nocturnal and daytime NVS. Patients with ventilatory muscle failure do not have unlimited ventilator-free breathing ability and require "ventilatory support," that is, up to continuous NVS to survive. This deserves further elucidation. Many patients with ventilatory insufficiency survive for years without ventilator use at the cost of increasingly severe hypercapnia, its associated symptoms and dangers, and a compensatory metabolic alkalosis that depresses the hypoxic and hypercapnic central ventilatory drive. The alkalosis allows the brain to accommodate to hypercapnia to avert acute ventilatory failure with its overt symptoms of obtundation, confusion, and coma. Indeed, studies show that when patients with neuromuscular disease re-breathe CO_2 they are unable to increase their ventilatory effort to sufficiently eliminate the CO_2 other than for a brief period of time. This is true although the pressure measured at the mouth at the initiation of a breath with the flow occluded at 100 ms (P100) is normal, indicating intact respiratory drive [1]. Peterson reported that the drive to breathe comes from under-stretching of lung stretch receptors as well as from hypoxia or hypercapnia [2].

The respiratory acidosis and metabolic alkalosis of patients with ventilatory insufficiency is corrected by NVS but often not by the usual noninvasive ventilation. This permits the kidneys to excrete excess bicarbonate ions. Once CO_2 is normalized because of the need to take bigger breaths to maintain normal $PaCO_2$ and blood pH levels, the ventilator user becomes short of breath when discontinuing ventilator use and, at least temporarily, can lose ventilator-free breathing ability. Breathing tolerance can be lost in supine, sitting, side lying, or all of the aforementioned positions. Thus, without ventilator use, the untreated patient with severe ventilatory muscle dysfunction and ventilatory insufficiency develops increasingly severe hypercapnia that can eventually result in coma from CO_2 narcosis or in ventilatory ("respiratory") arrest despite the absence of intrinsic lung disease. With NVS, patients with ventilatory muscle dysfunction and little or no measurable vital capacity (VC) can maintain normal alveolar ventilation, in some cases by using only nocturnal NVS, indefinitely, for as long as 65 years as seen in several of our patients. Thus, ventilatory ("respiratory") muscle failure can result in ventilatory failure but not necessarily respiratory failure, since both O_2 and CO_2 levels can be maintained within normal limits by using NVS and MIE to clear airway debris.

The combination of NVS and MIE can permit patients to avoid episodes of ARF or need for tracheostomy tubes despite total respiratory muscle paralysis and unmeasurable VCs. This can often be achieved by a telemedicine evaluation and is important because patients using or dependent on continuous NVS, as in many neuromuscular diseases (NMDs), have better long-term prognoses than patients who are not offered physical medicine interventions, who often cannot avoid episodes of ARF and resort to using tracheostomy mechanical ventilation (TMV). Patients can learn that ventilator unweanable patients with VPF who are intubated for acute on chronic ventilator failure can be extubated to continuous NVS and MIE without needing tracheotomies. Telemedicine permits clinicians expert in noninvasive ventilatory management to switch suboptimally managed patients using NIV to NVS and other complementary interventions (e.g., MIE) to relieve their symptoms of hypoventilation and spare their necks from tracheostomy tubes.

Preparation for the Telemedicine Visit

Telemedicine visits can take place with or without the presence of a home care respiratory therapists. Patients who have been pre-scribed portable ventilators such as the Trilogy™ (Respironics Inc., Murrysville, PA) or Astral™ (Stafford, TX) often have monthly visits by respiratory therapists to maintain the respiratory equipment. Patients who are symptomatic for VPF have often been prescribed portable ventilators to deliver bi-level PAP. For these patients, telemedicine visits can be arranged to coincide with the presence of the therapists who can bring four devices important for evaluation. These include a spirometer, peak flow meter, capnograph (end-tidal CO_2 monitor), and oximeter. Patients who cannot have a home care therapist present should be instructed to obtain a $7 oximeter and perhaps a $15 peak flows meter for the evaluation.

General Considerations

The room should be adequate to visualize the patient's body, especially the upper torso, and not just the face and head. It should be free of distractions and with adequate lighting. For the basics of optimal room setup, camera adjustment, space and positioning techniques for adequate examination, refer to Chap. 3.

Patient Interview

The patient history starts with a review of symptoms, including their beginning, duration, and concomitant diagnoses and other factors needed to differentiate primarily oxygenation impairment with hypoxemia from ventilation impairment on the basis of central hypoventilation from central respiratory controller hypoactivity, excessive work of breathing, restrictive lung disease, or respiratory muscle dysfunction and VPF. Patients with VPF often have a history of having had one or more pneumonias, respiratory hospitalizations, and intubations or even tracheostomy tube placements due to upper respiratory infections (URIs) developing into pneumonias and ARF because of ineffective CPF, often under 270 L/m. Patients without a history of asthma, obstructive pulmonary disease, wheezing, bronchiectasis, or other history of lung conditions are likely to have essentially pure VPF.

Symptoms of VPF and alveolar hypoventilation include:
Shortness of breath when supine (respiratory orthopnea)
Morning headaches
Fatigue
Daytime sleepiness
Difficulty concentrating
Depression
Loss of appetite

Anxiety
Sleep dysfunction and arousals
Nightmares
Shortness of breath
Irritability
Decreased libido
Urinary frequency
Weight loss
Muscle aches
Memory impairment
Nausea
Poor control of airway secretions
Symptoms of heart failure and leg swelling
Confusion, obtundation, or coma
Respiratory arrest

Physical Exam

For new patient referrals, the virtual visit can screen patients for pulmonary disease vs. VPF, for increased work of breathing, and shortness of breath who may benefit from urgent or emergent care at a hospital. On the other hand, patients with no history of lung or airways disease but who have generalized upper limb muscle weakness must be suspected of having VPF.

Inspection/Observation

- Examination should be with the patient sitting comfortably then supine.
- The patient's clothing should permit adequate visual assessment of the upper torso for accessory muscle use and tachypnea. Assess for increased work of breathing in the form of activation of sternocleidomastoid, latissimus dorsi, spinal, and neck extensors, which suggests excessive work of breathing.

- The skin, fingertips, and lips should be examined for bluish discoloration, which may be sign of poor oxygenation.
- The patient should be screened for neurologic changes (e.g., confusion, lack of coordination, lethargy).

These are important at the initial visit and at follow-up visits.

Specialized Testing

With the equipment described above, the physician informs the respiratory therapist to use the spirometer and peak flow meter to assess the VC in seated and supine positions, with any thoracic bracing on and off, for active and passive lung volume recruitment, glossopharyngeal breathing volumes, and manually assisted cough flows. Cough flows less than 300 L/m denote weak expiratory muscles and need for access to manually assisted coughing and possibly a CoughAssist™ for MIE to decrease risk of pneumonia and ARF. With a respiratory therapist present, both unassisted and assisted CPF can be measured at every patient visit via a peak flow meter.

All patients need pulse oximeters. A high heart rate can indicate hypercapnia, which means muscle impairment or increased work of breathing. An O_2 saturation less than 95% when awake may indicate hypercapnia, hypoventilation, airway secretions, or intrinsic lung disease. Pulse oximetry may need to be checked routinely. End-tidal CO_2 is determined with capnography. Since patients with VPF initially develop hypoventilation when reclining during sleep, VC supine along with CO_2 and O_2 saturation are important evaluation parameters for hypoventilation. Normally, the VC in sitting position is not more than 7.5% greater than when supine. When it is over 20% greater, the patient may be orthopneic and need NVS for better rest during sleep and for symptom relief.

It is prudent to recognize the pitfalls of interpreting polysomnograms, which diagnose central and obstructive apneas and hypopneas of sleep disordered breathing, rather than hypoventilation from VPF. Routine polysomnography was never designed to attribute the apneas and hypopneas to weak respiratory muscles rather than central or obstructive events. Thus, many patients are misdiagnosed, undertreated with low-span bi-level PAP, and remain symptomatic from hypoventilation. This is because polysomnography titrates down the apneas and hypopneas often without normalizing sleep CO_2 levels. Many of these orthopneic patients cannot sleep reclining even when using NIV. Thus, the telemedicine visit of patients, who continue to have symptoms of hypoventilation and cannot sleep supine using NIV, informs the clinician that the patient needs to be switched to NVS and possibly MIE when CPF are less than 300 L/m.

For patients without definitive symptoms, the physician may order sleep end-tidal CO_2 and O_2 saturation monitoring to be completed overnight at home. End-tidal CO_2 or transcutaneous CO_2 greater than 45 mmHg with the person awake is high and termed "hypercapnia." The hypercapnia is likely to be worse when sleeping. When sleep end-tidal CO_2 levels approach 50 mmHg and O_2 saturations frequently drop below 95% during sleep, a trial of sleep NVS is recommended, which can be ordered by the physician via telemedicine visit.

Indications for Treatment and Prescriptions

When specialized testing is unavailable, symptoms of fatigue, morning headaches, daytime drowsiness, persistent dyspnea, orthopnea, and possibly accessory muscle use, indicate the need for sleep NVS. Patients already using NIV need to be switched to bi-level PAP on NVS settings or switched from the passive ventilator circuit and vented nasal interfaces of bi-level PAP to active ventilator circuits and non-vented nasal interfaces using either volume or pressure assist-control settings without EPAP or PEEP. The NVS prescription is preferably volume-preset ventilation at 700–1400 mL volumes, back-up rate of 12 breaths/min, and FiO_2 of 21% with zero PEEP for patients who can close their glottises to hold consecutively delivered volumes for "air stacking" to deep lung volumes for active lung volume recruitment. The home care respiratory therapist, who delivers the equipment, works with the patient to determine the preferred settings between the ranges prescribed. NVS settings for patients who cannot air stack or who have excessive abdominal distension may trial pressure assist-control ventilation at full NVS settings of 19–22 cm H_2O and back-up rate of 12–14 breaths/min for patients with normal pulmonary compliance, but up to 50 cm H_2O pressure for the morbidly obese. These NVS settings can normalize blood gases and completely relieve respiratory symptoms around-the-clock and can be used indefinitely without any resort to tracheotomies even for rapidly weakening patients whose VCs decrease to unmeasurable levels and for patients with no ventilator-free breathing ability.

Patients whose unassisted CPF are below 300 L/m or who apparently have weak coughs, and a history of difficulty clearing airway debris, are informed that in the event of an upper respiratory tract infection or any difficulty clearing airway debris, they will need mechanical insufflation–exsufflation in the form of a CoughAssist™ prescribed by the physician. Mechanical insufflation–exsufflation is used at 50–60 cm H_2O pressures via oronasal or mouthpiece interface.

O_2 desaturation below 95% is caused by hypoventilation with hypercapnia, airway secretions, or lung disease. The oximetry feedback protocol, frequent use of MIE to clear airway congestion combined with NVS to recover fatigued respiratory muscles, is used to maintain or return O_2 saturation back to 95% or greater. If the congestion is not quickly cleared with the oximetry feedback protocol, atelectasis or pneumonia may develop, leading to further complications including ARF necessitating intubation. It is critical to clear airway mucus causing dyspnea in the setting of upper respiratory tract infections. Since adults over age 40 have few upper respiratory tract infections, the physician may prescribe a CoughAssist™ to be available on standby; when the patient needs it, a simple call to a reliable home care company for delivery can prevent severe respiratory complications. On the other hand, children with weak coughs may benefit from a CoughAssist™ in their homes for use during their relatively frequent upper respiratory tract infections to prevent pneumonia and ARF. Education and training in using oximetry for feedback as per the oximetry feedback protocol can be done by telemedicine visit with or without the presence of a respiratory therapist.

The oximetry feedback protocol is additionally used to prepare intubated and tracheostomized patients for extubation, and during post-extubation and post-decannulation. While not immediately relevant at the time of the telemedicine visit, the patients need to be informed that no patients with any neuromuscular disease other than classic ALS should ever require a tracheostomy tube for failing intubation if the patient is trained in the oximetry feedback protocol. No intubated patient needs to consent to having a tracheostomy tube placed other than some ALS patients with stridor from upper motor neuron disease [3].

Follow-Up

For patients with classic symptomology and VPF, those with improving symptoms should have respiratory parameters evaluated at each subsequent televisit, preferably in the presence of their home care respiratory therapist. Those without improving symptoms should be evaluated at an in-person visit. If the patient is unable to be connected with a home care respiratory therapist with access to a spirometer, peak flow meter, capnograph, and oximeter, then the patient should be brought into the office for in-person evaluation.

Conclusion/Summary

Patients with respiratory muscle weakness, severe obesity, high-level spinal cord injury, scoliosis, or Ondine's curse can benefit from NVS. Settings are prescribed as a range of volume 700–1500 mL and back-up rate 10–12 breaths/min, with the expert respiratory therapist determining the precise settings preferred by the patient. If volume-preset ventilation causes too much abdominal distension during sleep, it is switched to pressure control at 18–24 cm H_2O, which should be below the normal 25 cm H_2O integrity of the gastroesophageal sphincter. Primary and secondary settings can be programmed into the ventilator settings so that during the telemedicine visit, the patient can easily switch from one to the other. These settings optimally rest respiratory muscles and can provide up to full continuous NVS. The patient will find that he or she can again sleep supine and breathe day or night without shortness of breath. These settings normalize blood gases for all cooperative patients with VPF. Likewise, if CPF is determined to be ineffective by listening to them during the visit or by a history of repeated pneumonias, a CoughAssist™ is prescribed to be used at 50–60 cm H_2O pressures via oronasal or mouthpiece interfaces to clear secretions/aspirated material to avert ARF and intubation. There is much that can be accomplished by telemedicine visit for the patient with respiratory muscle weakness.

References

1. Baydur A. Respiratory muscle strength and control of ventilation in patients with neuromuscular disease. Chest. 1991;99:330–8.
2. Peterson WP, Barbalata L, Brooks CA, et al. The effect of tidal volumes on the time to wean persons with high tetraplegia from ventilators. Spinal Cord. 1999;37:284–8.
3. Bach JR. Noninvasive respiratory management of patients with neuromuscular disease. Ann Rehabil Med. 2017;41(4):1–20. https://doi.org/10.5535/arm.2017.41.4.519.

The Telemedicine Functional Assessment

14

Joseph Herrera, Andrew Beaufort, and Kaitlyn E. Wilkey

Chief Complaint: Functional Testing

Physical Exam

Functional testing is an important component to a thorough musculoskeletal examination of an entire limb or region. Essentially, incorporating functional testing allows for the provider to understand a patient's reflexive movement patterns that harbor or portend inefficient, pathologic neuromuscular tendencies.

Web-Based Goniometers

Accurate measurement of range of motion is vital to a thorough functional assessment as limitations in many joints, or even a sin-

---

J. Herrera
Department of Rehabilitation and Human Performance,
Mount Sinai Hospital, New York, NY, USA
e-mail: joseph.herrera@mountsinai.org

A. Beaufort (✉) · K. E. Wilkey
Department of Rehabilitation and Human Performance, Icahn School of Medicine at Mount Sinai, New York, NY, USA
e-mail: andrew.beaufort@mountsinai.org;
kaitlyn.wilkey@mountsinai.org; Wilkeyk8@rowan.edu

© The Author(s), under exclusive license to Springer Nature Switzerland AG 2023
M. Zakhary et al. (eds.), *Telemedicine for the Musculoskeletal Physical Exam*, https://doi.org/10.1007/978-3-031-16873-4_14

gle articulation, can result in observable differences in functional testing [1–4]. Web-based goniometers are helpful tools for providers to get reliable and accurate measurements of joint range of motion [5–9]. Efforts continue to be made in expanding their clinical utility and streamlining their use for telemedicine [7, 8].

Functional Assessments

Functional Assessment of the Upper Limb

Currently, there exists a dearth of validated functional physical capacity assessments for the shoulder, elbow, wrist, and hand that can be performed through a telemedicine visit. However, functional assessment of the upper limb should be pragmatic and consider the day-to-day challenges a patient is likely to face given the impairment of a particular joint or muscle group. A convenient addition to any musculoskeletal exam involving the upper extremities would include a grading system for the amount of functional range present in the limb.

Shoulder

Mannerkopi et al. devised a point system to assess, and trend, external rotation, internal rotation, and abduction of the shoulder across the midline [10]. With the patient sitting comfortably in a chair without arm rests have them perform the following movements separately, grading each separately based on their best effort. Additionally, in the sixth edition of *Orthopedic Physical Assessment*, Magee adds a third component to this functional test including adduction of the shoulder [11].

1. Bring the hand to the neck [10].
   (a) Fingers reach the posterior midline with shoulder fully abducted and externally rotated without wrist extension: 0 points.
   (b) Fingers reach the posterior midline without full shoulder abduction or external rotation: 1 point.
   (c) Fingers reach the neck, not the posterior midline: 3 points.
   (d) Fingers do not reach the neck: 4 points.

2. Bring the hand to the contralateral scapula (posteriorly) [10].
   (a) Fingers reach the scapula or 5 cm beneath it with full internal rotation: 0 points.
   (b) Fingers reach 6–15 cm below the scapula: 1 point.
   (c) Fingers reach the contralateral iliac crest: 2 points.
   (d) Fingers reach the buttock: 3 points.
   (e) Cannot bring hand behind the trunk: 4 points.
3. Bring the hand to the contralateral scapula (anteriorly) [12].
   (a) Hand reaches spine of contralateral scapula with full adduction without wrist flexion: 0 points.
   (b) Hand reaches spine of scapula with full adduction: 1 point.
   (c) Hand passes the midline of the trunk: 2 points.
   (d) Hand cannot pass the midline of the trunk: 3 points.

Assessing Functional Strength of the Shoulder

Strength testing in all planes of movement of the upper limbs can be clinically useful to identify localized deficits. Palmer and Epler proposed the following functional strength testing, Table 14.1:

Elbow

The majority of instability testing of the elbow requires stabilizing either the humerus or forearm during single plane movements [15]. Posterolateral instability of the elbow can present following injury to the lateral collateral ligament complex either through a traumatic event or dislocation [15–17]. Individuals will complain of snapping, locking, and catching about the elbow while it is extended and supinated. A 2006 publication by Regan et al. examined a proposed functional assessment for posterolateral rotatory instability [16].

Push-Up Test

We will describe two variations of the Push-Up Test [16, 17]. In order to perform this functional assessment, the patient must be able to perform a push-up ideally without a fulcrum of knees and lower leg resting on the ground [16, 17]. Patient is asked to supi-

Table 14.1 Assessing functional strength of the shoulder

Shoulder movement	Muscles involved	Functional	Functionally fair	Functionally poor	Non-functional
Forward flexion	Anterior deltoid, pectoralis major, biceps brachii, coracobrachialis	Lift 4–5 lb. weight	Lift 1–3 lb. weight	Lift arm weight	Cannot lift arm
Abduction	Middle deltoid, supraspinatus	Lift 4–5 lb. weight	Lift 1–3 lb. weight	Lift arm weight	Cannot lift arm
External rotation	Infraspinatus, teres minor, posterior deltoid, supraspinatus	Lift 4–5 lb. weight	Lift 1–3 lb. weight	Lift arm weight	Cannot lift arm
Internal rotation	Subscapularis, pectoralis major, latissimus dorsi, anterior deltoid, teres major	Lift 4–5 lb. weight	Lift 1–3 lb. weight	Lift arm weight	Cannot lift arm
Extension	Posterior deltoid, latissimus dorsi, teres major, long head of triceps, pectoralis major sternocostal portion	Lift 4–5 lb. weight	Lift 1–3 lb. weight	Lift arm weight	Cannot lift arm
Adduction	Pectoralis major, latissimus dorsi, teres major, coracobrachialis, infraspinatus, long head of triceps, anterior and posterior deltoid	Lift 4–5 lb. weight	Lift 1–3 lb. weight	Lift arm weight	Cannot lift arm
Elevation	Trapezius, levator scapulae, rhomboids	5–6 Repetitions	3–4 Repetitions	1–2 Repetitions	0 Repetitions
Push up	Compound movement: Pectoralis major, triceps brachii, anterior and middle deltoids	5–6 Repetitions	3–4 Repetitions	1–2 Repetitions	0 Repetitions

Sources: Palmer and Epler [13] and Brown et al. [14]

nate the extremity in question while maintaining the contralateral limb in usually push-up position (pronated forearm) [16, 17]. Patient performs a push-up followed by another push-up with upper limb supination [16, 17]. Reproduction of symptoms with supinated push-up rather than pronated is consistent with posterolateral rotatory instability [16, 17]. Alternatively, the test can be performed with the individual sitting on the ground with knees extended, extending the torso backward and supporting the body with their shoulder extended back with forearms maximally supinated [17, 18]. Patient attempts to lift their body, pushing up through both upper limbs and the feet as the only other point of contact [17, 18]. Patient then attempts to perform the same with forearms maximally pronated [17, 18]. Reproduction of symptoms with supinated push-up rather than pronated is consistent with posterolateral rotatory instability [17, 18]. The patient can perform this test while seated on a firm chair or surface.

Stand-Up Test
Patient begins seated [16]. Patient attempts to stand up placing the hands on the sitting surface with forearms maximally supinated [16]. Reproduction of symptoms, including pain, is considered a positive test [16].

Functional Assessment of the Lower Limb

Hip
Functional assessment of the lower limbs naturally require coordinated effort of multiple articulations including the hips, knees, and ankles. At the hip, functional testing can provide an adequate reflection of the patient's injury risk and pathologic movement patterns [19–22].

Maximum Depth Squat
Patient faces the camera at a distance where the both lower limbs can be fully visualized [23, 24]. The patient then assumes a reasonably athletic position (slight knee flexion, feet shoulder width apart) [23, 24]. Patient will then perform a double-legged body-

weight squat to their max depth after 2–3 warm-up attempts, if necessary [23, 24]. Careful attention should be paid to asymmetric movement at either of the major articulation [23, 24].

Single Leg Squat [25–30]
Patient faces the camera at a distance where both the lower limbs can be fully visualized. The patient then assumes a reasonably athletic position with feet shoulder width apart. Patient may use the upper extremity contralateral to the stance leg to balance. Patient will then perform a single-legged bodyweight squat to their max depth after 2–3 warm-up attempts, if necessary.

Single Leg Squat Variations [28]
If suspecting quadriceps dysfunction in the stance leg, it may be better elicited by asking the patient to extend the hip of the non-stance leg, bringing the limb largely behind the patient during the squat attempt. If there is concern of gluteal or hamstring pathology, patient may keep the non-stance leg in front of the stance leg or at the same level in order to elicit possible weakness or pain. History of stance leg ACL pathology should preclude use of the non-stance leg forward variation of the single leg squat as the diminished forward truncal lean is known to increase ACL forces during squatting.

Self-Paced Walk Test [31, 32]
Described with slight variations, we will suggest the most pragmatic approach with a level, obstacle-free corridor. Patient is asked to mark a spot 10 m (32.8 feet) away from the starting point. They will then reach this point and return for a total of 40 m. Their time to finish the task at a brisk but safe speed is recorded. Improvement greater than or equal to 0.2 m/s in performance is considered clinically impactful [31].

13 Meter Walk Test [19, 33]
Using a similar approach as the 50 Foot Walk Test, the patient is asked to select a single 52.6 foot stretch of level ground without obstacles. The patient will be asked to use a 1.5 m acceleration

phase and a 1.5 m deceleration phase at the beginning and the end of the 13 m walk, respectively. Performance on this functional test closely correlates with performance on the 6-Minute Walk Test, providing another option for patients who may have difficulty walking for 6 min. individuals who take longer to complete the 13 Meter Walk Test, walk a shorter distance on the 6-Minute Walk Test [19, 33, 34]. Furthermore, the brevity of this functional assessment enables one to measure the velocity of the patient and determine the ability to safely cross an intersection, measured at approximately >1.2 m/s [19, 35].

Timed Up and Go Test [36–39]
Patient starts from a seated position in a chair without armrests. The patient stands up and walks to a location 10 feet (3 m) directly in front of the chair and then returns to sitting in the chair. Patient's time is recorded and tracked. Studies have consistently indicated that higher TUG scores generally correlate with more pain, higher functional disability, and reduced HRQoL [39]. There is evidence suggesting that this functional assessment measure displayed moderate to strong evidence for positive ratings for both test-retest reliability and construct validity [40, 41]. Clinically, a reduction equal to or greater than 0.8, 1.4, and 1.2 s for the TUG indicates meaningful improvement in test performance [31].

Knee
Functional testing of the knee represents a confluence of balance, strength, proprioception, and core stability relying heavily on single leg hopping movements. Although challenging, single-legged hop tests have been found to have high reliability. As such it is critical to have minimum criteria to consider for functional assessment. Clark et al. proposed multiple criteria in their 2001 publication including: no pain, no effusion, no crepitus, full active range of motion (ROM) with terminal knee extension, symmetrical gait including climbing and descending stairs, and multiple single-legged balance measures [42]. It is worth considering most, if not all, of the listed criteria for embarking on a telemedicine functional assessment of the lower limbs, particularly the knees.

One-Legged Hop Test for Distance [43]

Choose a level, obstacle-free corridor. Measure distance covered by the patient's maximum hop using only one limb. Three times per leg alternating to either extremity each time. The average of all three attempts per leg is recorded [43]. Knee with ligamentous instability will have lower average on the three attempts that the uninjured extremity [43].

Timed One-Legged Hop Test [44–46]

Choose a level, obstacle-free corridor. Patient will measure 20 feet in a straight line. Once well demarcated, the patient will attempt to cover the 20 feet by hopping on one leg in the shortest amount of time safely possible. Patient then attempts with the contralateral limb.

Maximal Controlled Leap Test [47]

Choose a level, obstacle-free corridor. The patient then stands on the affected lower limb. The patient is then instructed to hops forward, landing on the contralateral leg without moving for 1 s at least [47]. The distance covered by the single leap is recorded and tracked [47].

Three Hop Test [44–46, 48]

Choose a level, obstacle-free corridor. Patient is instructed to hop forward on one leg three times in series. Total distance covered is measured. Patient then hops forward on the contralateral limb three times. Distance is compared between the injured and uninjured limb.

Ankle

Standing Balance [49–51]

Patient is asked to stand barefoot on a level surface. Patient assumes single leg stance with the hips level and eyes initially open for 10 s then closed for 10 s. Patient is observed for signs of failed balance (legs touched each other, the feet moved on the floor, the foot touches down, or the arms moved from their start position) or patient reports difficulty with balance. Failing to maintain balance for the 20 s test period on either laterality should prompt repeat assessment on the same extremity; repeat for the opposite foot. Patient with current suspected ankle sprain or history of ankle sprain have been found to exhibit positive Standing Leg Balance Testing [50].

Side Hop Test [52]
Performed in sneakers, the patient is asked to either create a line on the ground that is easily observed by both patient and provider. The patient is then asked to hop over the line in parallel (side hop) as many times prior to fatiguing. The number of side hops is then recorded and tracked over time. A study comparing multiple functional hopping tests of the ankle found that performance on the side hop correlated well to performance on other testing [52, 53]. This test can be modified by amplifying the width of the line used for lateral hopping to 30 cm width [53]. The patient can then be asked to jump laterally over and back, (considered one rep) for a total of 2 min. The examiner should record two attempts if possible and note the time for a single hop as well. Individuals with functional ankle instability, defined as reporting giving way sensation of the ankle during testing, will have difficulty performing this task with diminished number of hops compared to their uninjured extremity as well as longer length of time to complete a single hop [53].

Strength testing in all planes of movement of the ankle can be clinically useful to identify localized deficits. Palmer and Epler proposed the following functional strength testing, Table 14.2:

Functional Assessment of the Spine

Cervical Spine
Palmer and Epler described simple functional testing of the cervical spine to complement a targeted physical examination of the spine [55].

Table 14.2 Functional assessment of the lower limb

Ankle movement	Muscles involved	Functional	Functionally fair	Functionally poor	Non-functional
Single leg plantar flexion	Gastrocnemius, soleus, plantaris, flexor digitorum longus, peroneus longus, peroneus brevis, flexor hallucis longus, tibialis posterior	10–15 Repetitions	5–9 Repetitions	1–4 Repetitions	0 Repetitions
Single leg dorsi flexion	Tibialis anterior, extensor digitorum longus, extensor hallucis longus, peroneus tertius	10–15 Repetitions	5–9 Repetitions	1–4 Repetitions	0 Repetitions
Single leg inversion	Tibialis posterior, flexor digitorum longus, flexor hallucis longus, tibialis anterior, extensor hallucis longus	5–6 Repetitions	3–4 Repetition	1–2 Repetitions	0 Repetitions
Single leg eversion	Peroneus longus, peroneus brevis, peroneus tertius, extensor digitorum longus	5–6 Repetitions	3–4 Repetition	1–2 Repetitions	0 Repetitions
Toe flexion (seated)	Flexor digitorum longus, flexor hallucis longus, flexor digitorum brevis, flexor hallucis brevis, flexor accessorius (quadratus plantae), interossei, flexor digiti minimi brevis, lumbricals (metatarsophalangeal joints)	10–15 Repetitions	5–9 Repetitions	1–4 Repetitions	0 Repetitions
Toe extension (seated)	Extensor digitorum longus, extensor hallucis longus, extensor digitorum brevis, lumbricals (interphalangeal joints)	10–15 Repetitions	5–9 Repetitions	1–4 Repetitions	0 Repetitions

Adapted Sources: Palmer and Epler [13], Brown et al. [14] and Magee [54]

Supine
1. Neck flexion
    (a) At least three repetitions: fair functional strength.
    (b) 6–8 repetitions full functional strength.
2. Neck rotation
    (c) Hold for at least 10 s: fair functional strength.
    (d) Hold for 20–25 s: full functional strength.

Prone
1. Neck extension
    (a) Hold for at least 10 s: fair functional strength.
    (b) Hold for 20–25 s: full functional strength.

Side Lying
1. Lateral flexion
    (a) Hold for at least 10 s: fair functional strength.
    (b) Hold for 20–25 s: full functional strength.

Cervical Myelopathy
Patients with cervical compression myelopathy develop lower limb spasticity. Upper motor neuron weakness as well as positional sense disturbances (long tract signs) result in objective functional testing abnormalities when measured in series for an individual patient.

Simple Walking Test
Singh and Crockard described a Simple Walking Test [56]. Having measured a 15 m path void of any obstacles or uneven surfaces, the patient is asked to walk back and forth the full distance [56]. Examiner counts the number of steps and measures the time to complete the task safely [56].

Foot Tapping Test
Individuals with cervical myelopathy have been found to have difficulty with a simple foot tapping test [57]. Patient sits, preferably on a chair, with hips and knees flexed to 90° [57]. Patient is instructed to tap the sole of the foot as many times as they can in

10 s while keeping the heel planted on the ground [57]. The examiner records the number of foot taps [57]. FTT correlates well with other measures of function for individuals with suspected cervical myelopathy [57, 58].

(Ten Second) Step in Place Test [59]

Additionally, patients with cervical compressive myelopathy exhibit diminished ability to step in place due to long tract weakness [59]. The Ten second step test measures the individuals ability to bring their thigh parallel to the floor without holding onto any objects [59]. Patients with lower limb osteoarthritis or other confounding condition affecting the lower extremities would be excluded from this test [59]. The total number of steps with thighs parallel to the ground (with 90° hip and knee flexion) is counted [59]. The results of two separate efforts are averaged.

A Ten Second Step Test result of less than 12.8 is well correlated with the presence of cervical compressive myelopathy [59].

Lumbar Spine

Conditions related to the lumbar spine produce a broad range of signs and symptoms that can manifest during functional assessment [60]. There is ample evidence linking performance on simple functional tests with the presence of low back pain and related lumbar spine conditions [36, 40, 41, 61–64].

Repeat Sit to Stand Test [36, 64]

Starting from a seated position, patient is asked to rise to a standing position and then sit back down. Patient repeats five times while the examiner keeps time in seconds. A systematic review examining the level of evidence associated with physical capacity tests among subjects with low back pain found this functional assessment to be among the most well supported with strong retest reliability, construct validity, and responsiveness [40].

Timed Up and Go Test: refer to Functional Assessment of the Lower Limbs.

Repeat Trunk Flexion Test [36, 41, 65, 66]

Starting from a standing position facing forward, patient is asked to flex the trunk forward to limit of range of motion. This is repeated ten (10) times while the examiner keeps time in seconds. Authors recommend performing the test twice and tracking the average of the first and second attempt.

50 Foot Walk Test [36, 67]

From a standing position, patient walks 25 feet and then walks back. Examiner will record time to complete the task in seconds. Patient can perform this test on their own using a stopwatch and report results back to the physician. There is evidence suggesting that this functional assessment measure displayed moderate to strong evidence for positive ratings for both test–retest reliability and construct validity [40, 41].

5-Minute Walk Test [36, 67]

After choosing a hazard free and level walking setting, the patient is asked to walk as far as they can for 5 min and measure the distance [36, 67]. Use of smartphone-based pedometers and or GPS-based activity trackers will be helpful for this functional assessment. Performance can be trended over time. Timed walking tests have demonstrated clinical utility by adding to the quality of outcome measurement among individuals with chronic low back pain [67]. There is evidence suggesting that this functional assessment measure displayed moderate to strong evidence for positive ratings for both test–retest reliability and construct validity [40, 41].

Loaded Reach Test [36, 41, 63, 68]

Reaching with a load while standing is compromised in individuals with lower back pain. Patient stands parallel to a wall and while maintaining the heel in contact with the ground reaches forward with the nearest arm, shoulder flexed to 90° with elbow in full extension. The individual holds a weight below 4.5 kg (9.9 lbs) in the outstretched extremity during the reach attempt. Use of a mounted ruler can be helpful, if not separate measurements can be made at the starting point and furthest point reached.

References

1. Attias M, Chevalley O, Bonnefoy-Mazure A, De Coulon G, Cheze L, Armand S. Effects of contracture on gait kinematics: a systematic review. Clin Biomech (Bristol, Avon). 2016;33:103–10. https://doi.org/10.1016/j.clinbiomech.2016.02.017.
2. Campbell TM, Trudel G. Knee flexion contracture associated with a contracture and worse function of the contralateral knee: data from the osteoarthritis initiative. Arch Phys Med Rehabil. 2020;101(4):624–32. https://doi.org/10.1016/j.apmr.2019.11.018.
3. Murphy MT, Skinner TL, Cresswell AG, Crawford RW, Journeaux SF, Russell TG. The effect of knee flexion contracture following total knee arthroplasty on the energy cost of walking. J Arthroplasty. 2014;29(1):85–9. https://doi.org/10.1016/j.arth.2013.04.039.
4. Sotelo M, Eichelberger P, Furrer M, Baur H, Schmid S. Walking with an induced unilateral knee extension restriction affects lower but not upper body biomechanics in healthy adults. Gait Posture. 2018;65:182–9. https://doi.org/10.1016/j.gaitpost.2018.07.177.
5. Tanaka MJ, Oh LS, Martin SD, Berkson EM. Telemedicine in the era of COVID-19: the virtual orthopaedic examination. J Bone Jt Surg Am. 2020;102(12):e57. https://doi.org/10.2106/JBJS.20.00609.
6. Russell TG, Jull GA, Wootton R. Can the internet be used as a medium to evaluate knee angle? Man Ther. 2003;8(4):242–6. https://doi.org/10.1016/s1356-689x(03)00016-x.
7. Bruyneel AV. Smartphone applications for range of motion measurement in clinical practice: a systematic review. Stud Health Technol Inform. 2020;270:1389–90. https://doi.org/10.3233/SHTI200456.
8. Keogh JWL, Cox A, Anderson S, et al. Reliability and validity of clinically accessible smartphone applications to measure joint range of motion: a systematic review. PLoS One. 2019;14(5):e0215806. https://doi.org/10.1371/journal.pone.0215806.
9. Eble SK, Hansen OB, Ellis SJ, Drakos MC. The virtual foot and ankle physical examination. Foot Ankle Int. 2020;41(8):1017–26. https://doi.org/10.1177/1071100720941020.
10. Mannerkorpi K, Svantesson U, Carlsson J, Ekdahl C. Tests of functional limitations in fibromyalgia syndrome: a reliability study. Arthritis Care Res. 1999;12(3):193–9. https://doi.org/10.1002/1529-0131(199906)12:3<193::aid-art6>3.0.co;2-n.
11. Magee DJ. "Principles and concepts." Orthopedic physical assessment. 6th ed. Amsterdam: Elsevier Saunders; 2014. p. 1–83.
12. Magee DJ. "Shoulder." Orthopedic physical assessment. 6th ed. Amsterdam: Elsevier Saunders; 2014. p. 252–387.
13. Palmer ML, Epler M. Clinical assessment procedures in physical therapy. Philadelphia: J.B. Lippincott; 1990. p. 68–7.

14. Brown DP, et al. Musculoskeletal medicine. In: Cuccurullo SJ, editor. Physical medicine and rehabilitation board review. 4th ed. New York: Demos Medical; 2010. p. 149–76.
15. Montgomery KD, et al. Physical examination of the elbow. In: Malanga GA, Mautner K, editors. Musculoskeletal physical examination: an evidence-based approach. Amsterdam: Elsevier; 2017. p. 72–87.
16. Regan W, Lapner PC. Prospective evaluation of two diagnostic apprehension signs for posterolateral instability of the elbow. J Shoulder Elbow Surg. 2006;15(3):344–6. https://doi.org/10.1016/j.jse.2005.03.009.
17. Hsu SH, Moen TC, Levine WN, Ahmad CS. Physical examination of the athlete's elbow. Am J Sports Med. 2012;40(3):699–708. https://doi.org/10.1177/0363546511428869.
18. Magee DJ. "Elbow." Orthopedic physical assessment. 6th ed. Amsterdam: Elsevier Saunders; 2014. p. 406–7.
19. Mori B, Lundon K, Kreder H. 13-Metre walk test applied to the elderly with musculoskeletal impairment: validity study. Physiother Can. 2005;57(3):217–24. https://doi.org/10.3138/ptc.57.3.217.
20. Wahezi SE, et al. Telemedicine during COVID-19 and beyond: a practical guide and best practices multidisciplinary approach for the orthopedic and neurologic pain physical examination. Pain Physician. 2020;23(4S):S205–38.
21. Kivlan BR, Martin RL. Functional performance testing of the hip in athletes: a systematic review for reliability and validity. Int J Sports Phys Ther. 2012;7(4):402–12.
22. Lin YC, Davey RC, Cochrane T. Tests for physical function of the elderly with knee and hip osteoarthritis. Scand J Med Sci Sports. 2001;11(5):280–6. https://doi.org/10.1034/j.1600-0838.2001.110505.x.
23. Endo Y, Miura M, Sakamoto M. The relationship between the deep squat movement and the hip, knee and ankle range of motion and muscle strength. J Phys Ther Sci. 2020;32(6):391–4. https://doi.org/10.1589/jpts.32.391.
24. Lamontagne M, Kennedy MJ, Beaulé PE. The effect of cam FAI on hip and pelvic motion during maximum squat. Clin Orthop Relat Res. 2009;467(3):645–50. https://doi.org/10.1007/s11999-008-0620-x.
25. McGovern RP, Christoforetti JJ, Martin RL, Phelps AL, Kivlan BR. Evidence for reliability and validity of functional performance testing in the evaluation of nonarthritic hip pain. J Athl Train. 2019;54(3):276–82. https://doi.org/10.4085/1062-6050-33-18.
26. Lewis CL, Foch E, Luko MM, Loverro KL, Khuu A. Differences in lower extremity and trunk kinematics between single leg squat and step down tasks. PLoS One. 2015;10(5):e0126258. https://doi.org/10.1371/journal.pone.0126258.
27. Hatton AL, Kemp JL, Brauer SG, Clark RA, Crossley KM. Impairment of dynamic single-leg balance performance in individuals with hip chon-

dropathy. Arthritis Care Res (Hoboken). 2014;66(5):709–16. https://doi.org/10.1002/acr.22193.
28. Khuu A, Foch E, Lewis CL. Not all single leg squats are equal: a biomechanical comparison of three variations. Int J Sports Phys Ther. 2016;11(2):201–11.
29. Burnham JM, Yonz MC, Robertson KE, et al. Relationship of hip and trunk muscle function with single leg step-down performance: implications for return to play screening and rehabilitation. Phys Ther Sport. 2016;22:66–73. https://doi.org/10.1016/j.ptsp.2016.05.007.
30. McGovern RP, Martin RL, Christoforetti JJ, Kivlan BR. Evidence-based procedures for performing the single leg squat and step-down tests in evaluation of non-arthritic hip pain: a literature review. Int J Sports Phys Ther. 2018;13(3):526–36.
31. Wright AA, Cook CE, Baxter GD, Dockerty JD, Abbott JH. A comparison of 3 methodological approaches to defining major clinically important improvement of 4 performance measures in patients with hip osteoarthritis. J Orthop Sports Phys Ther. 2011;41(5):319–27. https://doi.org/10.2519/jospt.2011.3515.
32. Kennedy DM, Stratford PW, Wessel J, et al. Assessing stability and change of four performance measures: a longitudinal study evaluating outcome following total hip and knee arthroplasty. BMC Musculoskelet Disord. 2005;6:3. https://doi.org/10.1186/1471-2474-6-3.
33. ATS Committee on Proficiency Standards for Clinical Pulmonary Function Laboratories. ATS statement: guidelines for the six-minute walk test [published correction appears in Am J Respir Crit Care Med. 2016;193(10):1185]. Am J Respir Crit Care Med. 2002;166(1):111–7. https://doi.org/10.1164/ajrccm.166.1.at1102.
34. Rikli R, Jones C. The reliability and validity of a 6-minute walk test as a measure of physical endurance in older adults. J Aging Phys Act. 1998;6(4):363–75. https://doi.org/10.1123/japa.6.4.363.
35. Hoxie RE, Rubenstein LZ. Are older pedestrians allowed enough time to cross intersections safely? J Am Geriatr Soc. 1994;42(3):241–4. https://doi.org/10.1111/j.1532-5415.1994.tb01745.x.
36. Simmonds MJ, Olson SL, Jones S, et al. Psychometric characteristics and clinical usefulness of physical performance tests in patients with low back pain. Spine (Phila Pa 1976). 1998;23(22):2412–21.
37. Podsiadlo D, Richardson S. The timed "Up & Go": a test of basic functional mobility for frail elderly persons. J Am Geriatr Soc. 1991;39(2):142–8. https://doi.org/10.1111/j.1532-5415.1991.tb01616.x.
38. Jakobsson M, Brisby H, Gutke A, Lundberg M, Smeets R. One-minute stair climbing, 50-foot walk, and timed up-and-go were responsive measures for patients with chronic low back pain undergoing lumbar fusion surgery. BMC Musculoskelet Disord. 2019;20(1):137. https://doi.org/10.1186/s12891-019-2512-5.

39. Gautschi OP, Joswig H, Corniola MV, et al. Pre- and postoperative correlation of patient-reported outcome measures with standardized Timed Up and Go (TUG) test results in lumbar degenerative disc disease. Acta Neurochir. 2016;158(10):1875–81. https://doi.org/10.1007/s00701-016-2899-9.
40. Jakobsson M, Gutke A, Mokkink LB, Smeets R, Lundberg M. Level of evidence for reliability, validity, and responsiveness of physical capacity tasks designed to assess functioning in patients with low back pain: a systematic review using the COSMIN standards. Phys Ther. 2019;99(4):457–77. https://doi.org/10.1093/ptj/pzy159.
41. Denteneer L, Van Daele U, Truijen S, De Hertogh W, Meirte J, Stassijns G. Reliability of physical functioning tests in patients with low back pain: a systematic review. Spine J. 2018;18(1):190–207. https://doi.org/10.1016/j.spinee.2017.08.257.
42. Clark NC. Functional performance testing following knee ligament injury. Phys Ther Sport. 2001;2:101.
43. Strobel M, Stedtfeld HW. Stress roentgen study of the knee joint—an evaluation of status. Unfallchirurg. 1986;89(6):272–9.
44. Noyes FR, Barber SD, Mangine RE. Abnormal lower limb symmetry determined by function hop tests after anterior cruciate ligament rupture. Am J Sports Med. 1991;19(5):513–8. https://doi.org/10.1177/036354659101900518.
45. Barber SD, Noyes FR, Mangine RE, McCloskey JW, Hartman W. Quantitative assessment of functional limitations in normal and anterior cruciate ligament-deficient knees. Clin Orthop Relat Res. 1990;255:204–14.
46. Booher LD, Hench KM, Worrell TW, et al. Reliability of three single-leg hop tests. J Sport Rehabil. 1993;2:165–70.
47. Juris PM, Phillips EM, Dalpe C, Edwards C, Gotlin RS, Kane DJ. A dynamic test of lower extremity function following anterior cruciate ligament reconstruction and rehabilitation. J Orthop Sports Phys Ther. 1997;26(4):184–91. https://doi.org/10.2519/jospt.1997.26.4.184.
48. Hopper DM, Goh SC, Wentworth LA, et al. Test–retest reliability of knee rating scales and functional hop tests one year following anterior cruciate ligament reconstruction. Phys Ther Sport. 2002;3:10–8.
49. Freeman MAR, Dean MRE, Hanham IWF. The etiology and prevention of functional instability of the foot. J Bone Jt Surg Br. 1965;47:678–85.
50. Trojian TH, McKeag DB. Single leg balance test to identify risk of ankle sprains. Br J Sports Med. 2006;40(7):610–3. https://doi.org/10.1136/bjsm.2005.024356.
51. Eechaute C, Vaes P, Duquet W. The dynamic postural control is impaired in patients with chronic ankle instability: reliability and validity of the multiple hop test. Clin J Sport Med. 2009;19(2):107–14. https://doi.org/10.1097/JSM.0b013e3181948ae8.

52. Greisberg J, Gould P, Vosseller JT, et al. Performance function tests in assessing ankle fitness. J Am Acad Orthop Surg Glob Res Rev. 2019;3(1):e096. https://doi.org/10.5435/JAAOSGlobal-D-18-00096.
53. Caffrey E, Docherty CL, Schrader J, Klossner J. The ability of 4 single-limb hopping tests to detect functional performance deficits in individuals with functional ankle instability. J Orthop Sports Phys Ther. 2009;39(11):799–806. https://doi.org/10.2519/jospt.2009.3042.
54. Magee DJ. "Lower leg, ankle, and foot." Orthopedic physical assessment. 6th ed. Amsterdam: Elsevier Saunders; 2014. p. 888–980.
55. Palmer ML, Epler M. Clinical assessment procedures in physical therapy. Philadelphia: J.B. Lippincott; 1990. p. 181–2.
56. Singh A, Crockard HA. Quantitative assessment of cervical spondylotic myelopathy by a simple walking test. Lancet. 1999;354(9176):370–3. https://doi.org/10.1016/S0140-6736(98)10199-X.
57. Numasawa T, Ono A, Wada K, et al. Simple foot tapping test as a quantitative objective assessment of cervical myelopathy. Spine (Phila Pa 1976). 2012;37(2):108–13. https://doi.org/10.1097/BRS.0b013e31821041f8.
58. Enoki H, Tani T, Ishida K. Foot tapping test as part of routine neurologic examination in degenerative compression myelopathies: a significant correlation between 10-sec foot-tapping speed and 30-m walking speed. Spine Surg Relat Res. 2019;3(3):207–13.
59. Yukawa Y, Kato F, Ito K, et al. "Ten second step test" as a new quantifiable parameter of cervical myelopathy. Spine (Phila Pa 1976). 2009;34(1):82–6. https://doi.org/10.1097/BRS.0b013e31818e2b19.
60. Cox ME, Asselin S, Gracovetsky SA, et al. Relationship between functional evaluation measures and self-assessment in nonacute low back pain. Spine (Phila Pa 1976). 2000;25(14):1817–26. https://doi.org/10.1097/00007632-200007150-00013.
61. Vachalathiti R, Sakulsriprasert P, Kingcha P. Decreased functional capacity in individuals with chronic non-specific low back pain: a cross-sectional comparative study. J Pain Res. 2020;13:1979–86. https://doi.org/10.2147/JPR.S260875.
62. Simmonds MJ, Claveau Y. Measures of pain and physical function in patients with low back pain. Physiother Theory Pract. 1997;13(1):53–65. https://doi.org/10.3109/09593989709036448.
63. Staartjes VE, Beusekamp F, Schröder ML. Can objective functional impairment in lumbar degenerative disease be reliably assessed at home using the five-repetition sit-to-stand test? A prospective study. Eur Spine J. 2019;28(4):665–73. https://doi.org/10.1007/s00586-019-05897-3.
64. Marras WS, Parnianpour M, Ferguson SA, et al. The classification of anatomic- and symptom-based low back disorders using motion measure models. Spine (Phila Pa 1976). 1995;20(23):2531–46. https://doi.org/10.1097/00007632-199512000-00013.

65. Marras WS, Wongsam PE. Flexibility and velocity of the normal and impaired lumbar spine. Arch Phys Med Rehabil. 1986;67(4):213–7.
66. Harding VR, Williams AC, Richardson PH, et al. The development of a battery of measures for assessing physical functioning of chronic pain patients. Pain. 1994;58(3):367–75. https://doi.org/10.1016/0304-3959(94)90131-7.
67. Duncan PW, Weiner DK, Chandler J, Studenski S. Functional reach: a new clinical measure of balance. J Gerontol. 1990;45(6):M192–7. https://doi.org/10.1093/geronj/45.6.m192.
68. Duncan PW, Studenski S, Chandler J, Prescott B. Functional reach: predictive validity in a sample of elderly male veterans. J Gerontol. 1992;47(3):M93–8. https://doi.org/10.1093/geronj/47.3.m93.

Index

A
Abduction, 84
Acetaminophen, 60
Achilles tendon palpation, 164
Achilles tendon reflex, 169
Adult spinal deformity, 54
Amputation, 122
Anatomic maneuver, 168
Ankle dorsiflexion, 129
Anterior drawer test, 170
Anterior talofibular ligament laxity, 170
Apley grind test, 140
Apley scratch test, 83
Axial back pain, 52

B
Babinski reflex, 59
Bicep's tendinopathy, 97–98
Bluetooth-enabled sensors, 8
Bone injuries, 133
Breathing tolerance, 186

C
Calcaneal palpation, 164
Calf palpation, 164
Carpal tunnel syndrome, 119, 120
Cervical myelopathy, 205
Chair push-up test, 95
Chronic pain, 53
Chronic ventilatory insufficiency, 184
Cobb angles, 54, 61
Coleman block test, 173
Computer tomography (CT), 88
Continuous positive airway pressure (CPAP), 184
Costovertebral pain, 56
CoughAssist™, 190, 192
COVID-19 world pandemic, 3
Cubital tunnel syndrome, 99
Current procedural terminology (CPT) codes, 12

D
Degenerative disc disease, 54
DeQuervain's tenosynovitis, 118
Dermatomyositis (DM), 28
Dermatomyositis/polymyositis, 31
Disc herniations, 55
Disease-modifying antirheumatic drugs (DMARDs), 32
Down syndrome, 45
Drop-arm test, 85
Duck walk (Childress test), 141
Dynamic radiographs, 61

E
Elbow dislocation, 102
Elbow flexion, 94
Elbow instability, 101
Elson's test, 113
Empty can test, 85
Exercise tolerance, 33
Extension, 84
External rotation, 84, 128

F
50 foot walk test, 207
5 minute walk test, 207
Flexion, 84
Flexion, abduction, external rotation of the hip (FABER), 129
Flexor tenosynovitis, 118
FOOSH injury, 110, 120
Foot and ankle exam
  chief complaint and history of present illness
    initial set-up, 161
    inspection, 161, 162
    neurologic and vascular examination, 166
    pain, 160
    palpation, 162
    reflex testing, 167
    strength testing, 166, 167
    swelling, 160
  differential diagnosis, 177
  followup, 181
  management and treatment, 177, 179
  red flags, 179
  seated special tests, 169, 170, 172
  standing/walking special tests, 173, 176
Foot tapping test, 205–206
Functional assessment
  of lower limb, 199, 200
  physical exam, 195
  of spine, 203, 206
  of upper limb, 196, 199
  web based goniometers, 196

G
Gait assessment, 175
General telemedicine exam
  chief complaint/patient history, 23, 24
  complications/red flags, 34
  dermatomyositis (DM), 28
  differential diagnosis, 27
  inspection/observation, 24, 25
  management/treatment, 31–33
  Marfan syndrome, 28
  palpation, 26, 27
  physical exam, 24
  rheumatic fever, 30, 31
  spondyloarthropathies, 29
  systemic lupus erythematosus (SLE), 28
Global Burden of Disease studies (GBD), 5

H
Hawkins test, 86
Health data, 1
High pressure injection injury, 121
Hip abduction, 127
Hip adduction, 127
Hip flexion, 127
Hoffman's sign, 59
Hop test, 176
Hypercapnia, 191
Hyperkyphosis, 54

I
Ibuprofen, 60
Internal rotation, 84, 128
Intra-articular hip pathologies, 133

J
Jersey finger, 116
Joint dislocations, 180
Joint instability, 102

Index

K
Kleiger's test, 172–174
Knee alignment, 126
Knee extension, 128

L
Lacerations, 111, 112
Lateral epicondylitis (tennis elbow), 96, 99, 102
Lateral malleolus palpation, 164
L4-5 nerve function, 176
Lisfranc fracture, 180
Loaded reach test, 207
Lower extremity muscle activation, 9

M
Mallet finger, 117
Marfan syndrome, 28, 31
Maximal controlled leap test, 202
Maximum depth squat, 199–200
Mechanical insufflation-exsufflation (MIE), 183, 192
Medial ankle sprain, 172–173
Medial epicondylitis (Golfer's elbow), 96, 98, 101
Medial malleolus palpation, 164
Metacarpophalangeal ulnar ligament rupture, 115
Metatarsal squeeze, 172, 173
Modified Stinchfield test, 130
Morton's/interdigital neuroma, 172
Moterum application, 10
Muscle strength, 85
Muscle strength testing, 51

N
Naproxen, 60
Navicular palpation, 164
Nerve entrapment injuries, 133
Neurovascular examination, 109
Noninvasive ventilatory support (NVS), 183

O
O'Brien's test, 86–87
Olecranon bursitis, 100
One-legged squat, 141
Open fracture, 121
Osteochondritis dissecans, 97
O_2 desaturation, 192
Oximetry feedback protocol, 193

P
Palpation, 83, 137
Patellar compression test, 139
Popeye sign, 102
Posterior impingement, 100
Posterior interroseus nerve syndrome, 100
PRICE protocol, 178
Prone provocative testing, 140
Prone stork test, 76
Pulmonary function, 55

R
Radial tunnel syndrome, 99
Radicular pain, 53, 55
Range of motion (ROM) testing, 83–84, 108, 137, 165
Referred pain, 53
Reflex testing, 52, 138, 146, 167
Remote patient monitoring
  barriers of, 11
  billing and coding legislation, 12
  defined, 1
  and MSK, 3, 5
  for musculoskeletal patient, 5, 6
    functional mobility, 10
    inspection, 6
    pain, 7
    palpation, 8
    range of motion, 7
    sensation, 9
    strength, 8, 9
  technology utilized, 10
  telemedicine/video visit, 2, 3, 11
Repeat trunk flexion test, 207

Resisted hip adduction, 130
Respiratory acidosis, 186
Respiratory muscle dysfunction
  follow-up, 193
  general considerations, 188
  patient interview, 188, 189
  physical exam, 189, 190
  preparation for telemedicine visit, 187
  specialized testing, 190, 191
  treatment and prescriptions, 191, 193
Retroperitoneal bleeding, 59
Rheumatic fever, 30, 31
Rheumatoid arthritis, 45
Rotator cuff, 82

S

Scaphoid fracture, 110
Scaphoid waist, 111
Scapular stability, 82
Scarf test, 86
Scheuermann disease, 55
Seated provocative testing, 140
Seated slump test, 130
Self paced walk test, 200
Sensation testing, 52, 74, 138, 144
Septic arthritis, 156
Side hop test, 203
Single foot tiptoe, 167
Single leg hop test, 131
Single leg squat, 200
Single leg squat variations, 200
Slump test, 75
Soft tissues injuries, 132
Speed's test, 86
Spondyloarthropathies, 29, 32
Spondylosis, 56
Spurling's neck compression test, 44
Spurling's test, 87
Standing provocative testing, 148
Standing push-up test, 85
Staphylococcal infections, 57

Static joint stability, 81
Strength assessment, 166
Strength testing, 138, 147
Supine provocative testing, 139
Systemic lupus erythematosus (SLE), 28

T

Talar instability, 170
Telemedicine cervical spine exam
  chief complaint/patient history, 39, 49
  in children, 45
  complications/red flags, 46
  differential diagnosis, 45–46, 52, 53, 55, 57, 59
  Down syndrome, 45
  L'hermitte's test, 44
  management/treatment, 46
    complications/red flags, 63
    follow up, 63
    mechanical, 60
    non-mechanical and visceral causes, 62
  physical exam
    active range of motion, 51
    initial setup, 50
    inspection, 40, 50
    muscle strength, 42, 43
    neurological examination, 51, 52
    palpation, 41, 51
Telemedicine cervical spine exam (*cont.*)
    range of motion, 41
    reflexes, 43
    sensation testing, 43
  rheumatoid arthritis, 45
  shoulder abduction test, 44
  special consideration, 59
  Spurling's neck compression test, 44
Telemedicine elbow exam

Index

biceps tendon tear (orthoinfo), 92
   chief complaint/patient history, 91
      inspection/observation, 92
      physical exam, 92
   complications/red flags, 102
   considerations for certain populations, 96
   differential diagnosis, 97
   elbow instability, 101
   lateral elbow pain, 99
   management/treatment, 101, 102
   neurological examination, 95
   posterior elbow pain, 100

Telemedicine hand and wrist exam
   chief complaint/patient history, 105
   complications/red flags, 121
   differential diagnosis
      lacerations, 111, 112, 115, 116, 119
      scaphoid fracture, 110
   follow up, 123
   inspection/observation, 107
   management/treatment, 120
   neurovascular examination, 109
   palpation, 107, 108
   physical exam, 106
   range of motion, 108
   special considerations, 119

Telemedicine hip exam
   chief complaint/patient history, 125
   complications/red flags, 133
   differential diagnosis, 131
   management/treatment, 132
   physical exam
      gait, 127
      inspection, 126
      muscle testing, 128
      palpation, 128
      range of motion, 127
      sensation, 129
      set-up, 126
   special considerations, 132
   special tests, 129, 130

Telemedicine knee exam
   complications and red flags, 156
   differential diagnoses, 154
   follow-up, 157
   history, 135, 136
   management and treatment, 155
   physical exam, 136, 138, 141, 143, 148
   special consideration, 155

Telemedicine lumbar spine exam
   active range of motion (ROM), 70
   extensor hallucis longus, 73
   follow up, 78
   gait, 71
   gastrocnemius-soleus, 73
   gluteus medius, 73
   history, 67
   inspection, 69, 70
   muscle strength testing, 71
   palpation, 70
   physical exam, 68
   psoas, 72
   quadricep strength, 72
   reflex testing, 73, 74
   sensation testing, 74
   special considerations, 78
   special testing
      Ely's test, 76
      Kemp's test, 75
      modified Gaenslen's test, 77
      prone stork test, 76
      reverse straight leg raise, 76
      seated straight leg raise, 74
      seated/supine FABER, 75
      slump test, 75
      standing stork test, 75
      supine FAIR, 77
      supine straight leg raise, 77
      Thomas test, 78
   tibialis anterior, 72

Telemedicine maneuver, 168
Telemedicine shoulder exam
 complications/red flags, 88
 differential diagnosis, 87
 follow-up, 89
 history, 82
 management/treatment, 87
 physical examination, 82, 85
 special test, 85
Thessaly test, 141
13 meter walk test, 200–201
30-second chair stand test (30s-CST), 10
Three hop test, 202
Timed up and go test (iTUG), 10, 201
Tiptoe walk, 175
Tracheostomy mechanical ventilation (TMV), 187
Transverse myelitis, 58
Triceps tendinopathy, 100
Two-legged squat, 141

U
Ulnar collateral ligament injury, 98
Upper respiratory infections (URIs), 188

V
Valgus stress test, 140
Varus stress test, 140
Vascular compromise, 180
Vascular Injury, 122
Velcro straps, 8
Ventilatory muscle failure, 185
Vertebral augmentation procedures, 61
Vertical surface dorsiflexed, 167
Video visit preparation and patient education
 after visit, 19
 clothing, 18
 during visit, 19
 helpful objects, 19
 ideal space, 18
 patient education, 20, 21
 visual and auditory quality, 18

W
Wearable sensors, 2
Web based goniometer, 94, 196

Y
Yergason's test, 86

GPSR Compliance

The European Union's (EU) General Product Safety Regulation (GPSR) is a set of rules that requires consumer products to be safe and our obligations to ensure this.

If you have any concerns about our products, you can contact us on ProductSafety@springernature.com

In case Publisher is established outside the EU, the EU authorized representative is:

Springer Nature Customer Service Center GmbH
Europaplatz 3
69115 Heidelberg, Germany

Batch number: 08823212

Printed by Printforce, the Netherlands